THE BOOK OF MATCHA

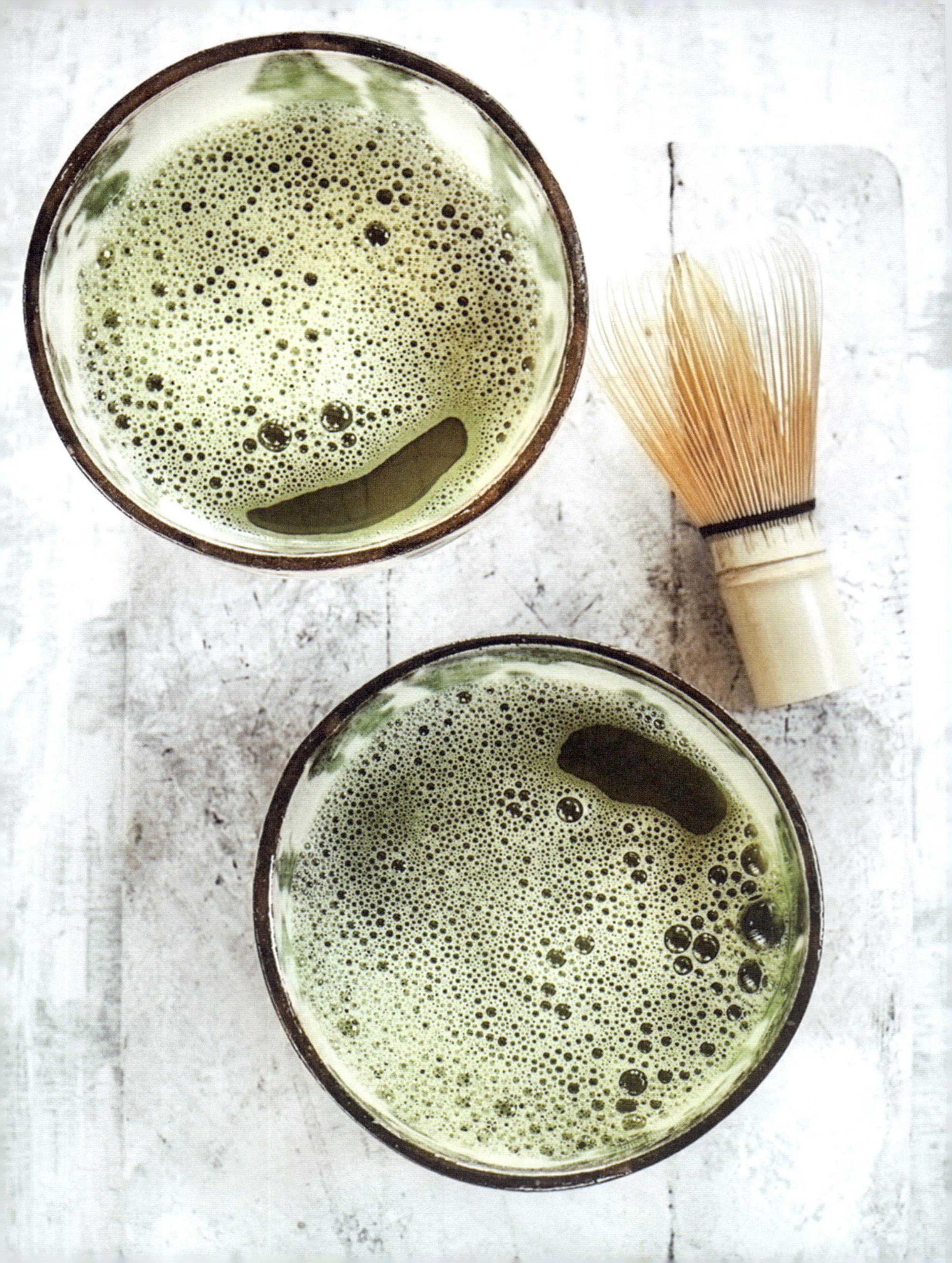

THE BOOK OF MATCHA

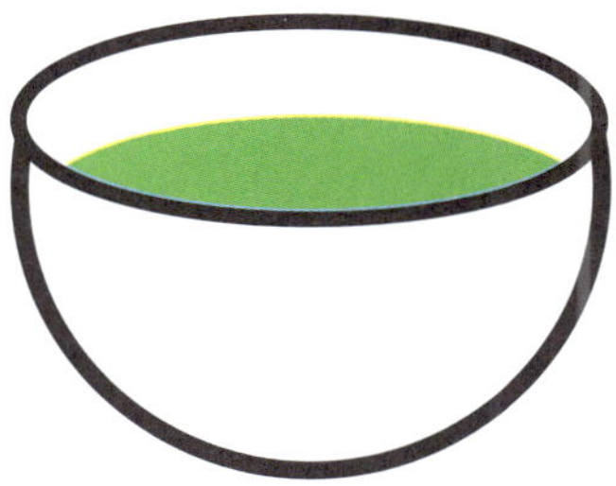

WHITE LION
PUBLISHING

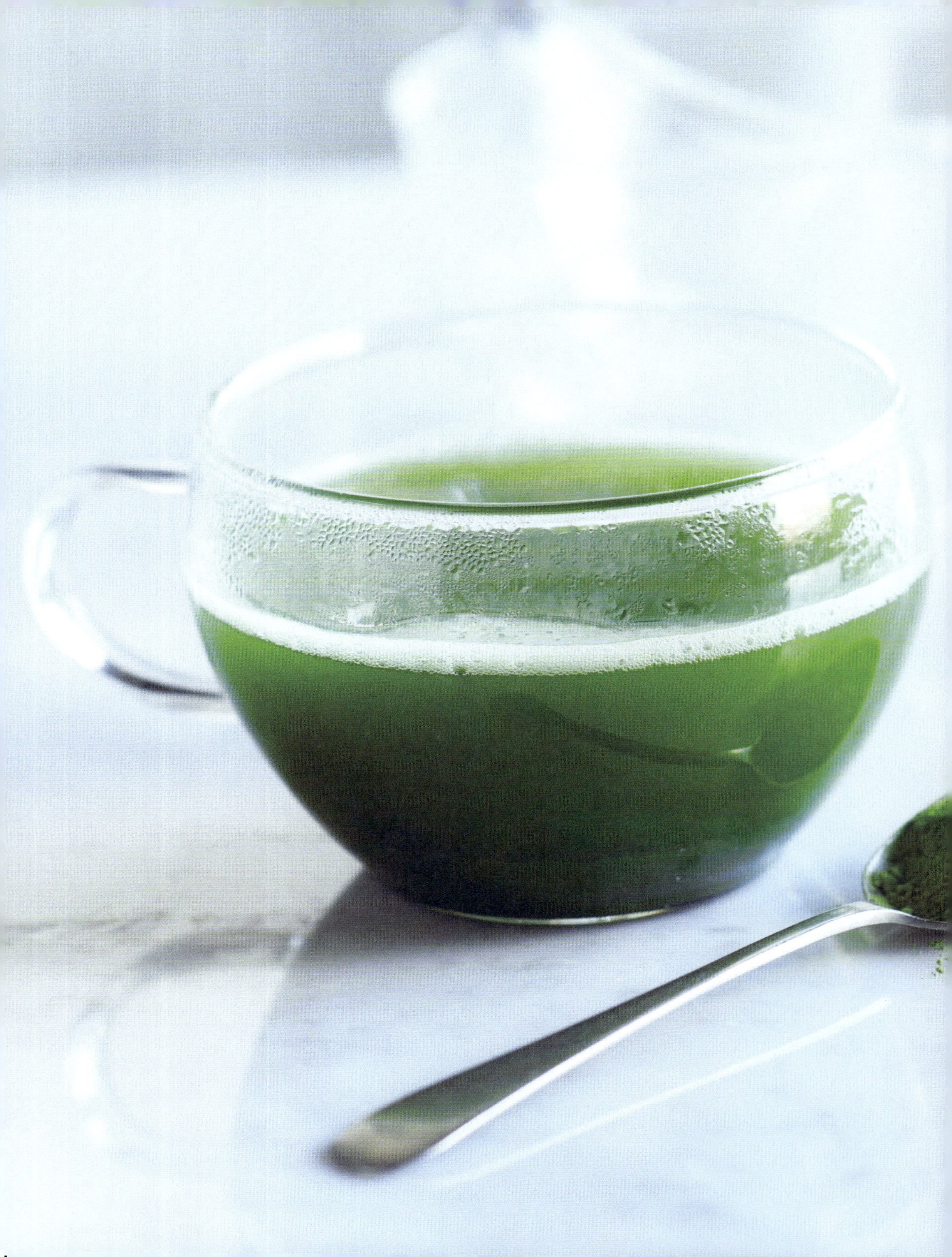

Contents

6 The history of matcha
20 The production of matcha
32 The health benefits
42 Matcha today
52 Matcha recipes
58 Drinks
72 Breakfast
92 Snacks
108 Main meals
132 Bakes
150 Desserts

170 Index
174 Acknowledgements

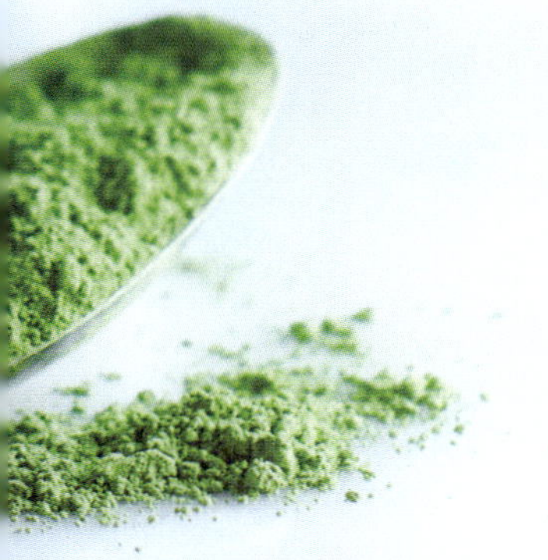

The history of matcha

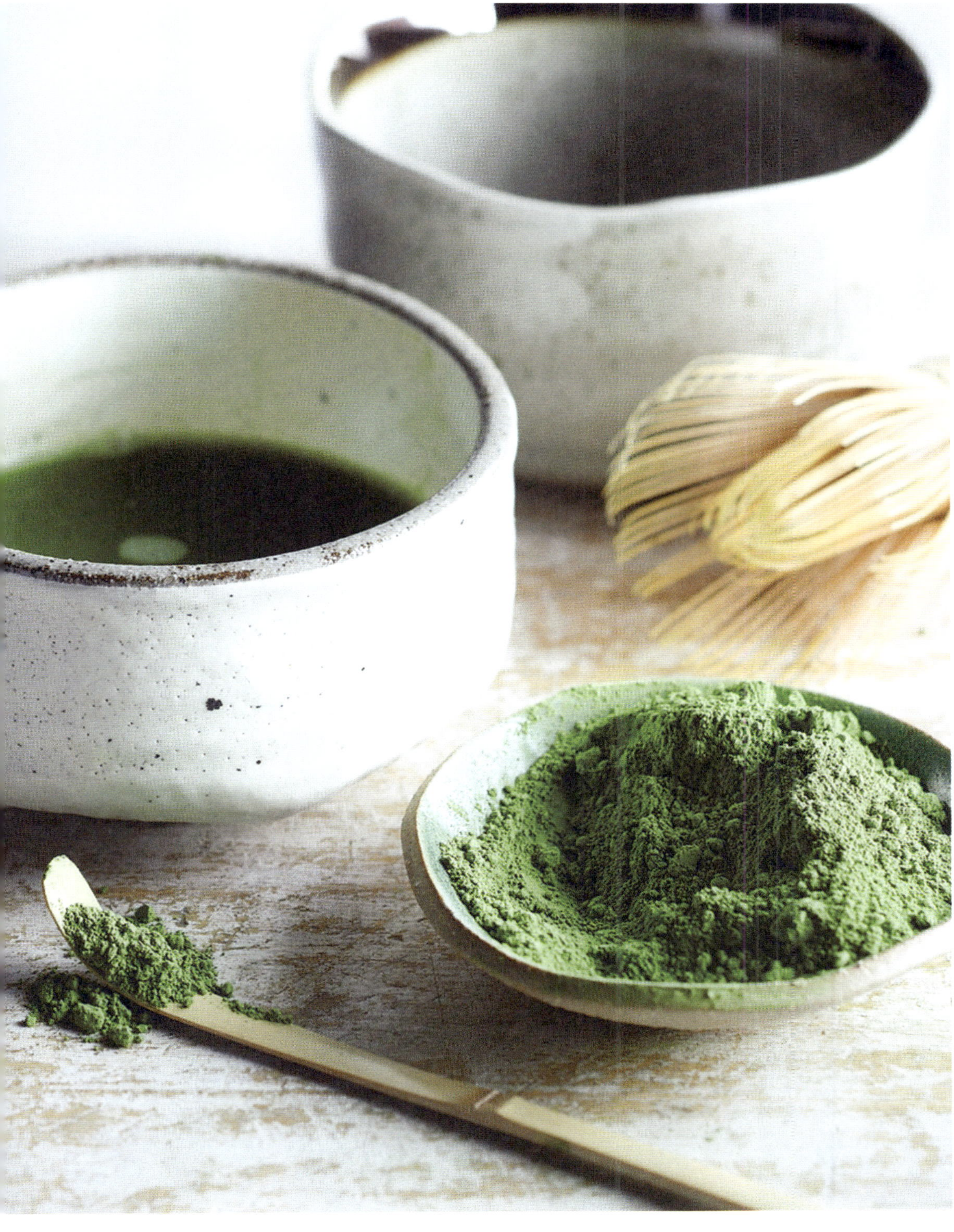

Matcha's origins

Although you may have only recently discovered matcha – the super-concentrated 100 per cent green tea powder – it is nothing new. Matcha has been drunk in Japan since the 12th century, and before that in China. Although the Japanese are considered to be the masters of matcha, key elements of matcha production originated in China.

In China, drinking green tea was commonplace in the 8th century, and the tradition of steaming and drying green tea into bricks was widespread. Then the Chinese Zen (Chan) monks got involved. They broke off chunks from the brick and ground it into a very fine powder using a pestle and mortar, before whisking the powder with hot water in a large bowl to make their green tea. The whisking of the ground green tea leaves became a key part of the Zen Buddhist daily ritual.

Matcha came to Japan when Myoan Eisai, a big-hitting Japanese monk, discovered ground green tea leaves while travelling in China in the late 1180s to study Zen Buddhist meditation. In love with China, Zen Buddhism and ground green tea leaves, he returned to Japan in 1191 with a few tea plant seeds. He then began a very successful one-monk campaign to popularize Zen Buddhism within Japan and promote the consumption of matcha, which he believed was vital for meditation.

Myoan Eisai (1141–1215), Zen Master

Eisai was the founder of the Rinzai sect of Zen Buddhism and was known as a great reformer. Not only did he bring tea plant seeds from China, he also wrote widely of the health benefits of tea and matcha. His book Kissa Yojoki, *which means 'drinking tea for health', was published in 1211 and was the first book about tea to be published in Japan. The first line reads: 'Tea is the ultimate mental and medical remedy and has the ability to make one's life more full and complete'.*

Eisai believed the Chinese lived a long and healthy life due to their consumption of tea and its medicinal properties, and encouraged the Japanese to take on this tea-drinking habit.

> **MATCHA IS 'THE ELIXIR OF THE IMMORTALS'**
> EISAI

The Chinese moved on to other teas, including pu-erh, oolong and black tea (which they call 'red tea'). Meanwhile, in Japan, the popularity of green tea developed further, with matcha soon becoming an intrinsic part of Japanese life.

MATCHA GROWS IN POPULARITY

Zen monasteries in Japan embraced the matcha movement as the monks found that the long periods of meditation were easier with matcha inside. The L-theanine (whether they knew it or not) kept them calm and alert for long periods of time. See also The health benefits (page 32).

Enjoying matcha became part of the cultural tradition and the artistic life of Japan. Those who enjoyed poetry, music and high society activities also enjoyed the luxurious (and expensive) matcha. As the Samurai class (early Japanese nobility), aristocrats and intellectuals began to truly understand and appreciate matcha, it grew in popularity over

The Japanese Tea Masters

Tea masters spend years learning and perfecting the spiritual and ritual practices of the tea ceremony. In the 15th and 16th centuries there were a number of important grand tea masters:

Ikkyu Sojun (1394–1481)
A Japanese Zen Buddhist priest, poet and tea master, he was one of the great influencers. Credited with an edgy and eccentric approach to Buddhism, he was respected for his great tea practice.

Murato Shuko (1422–1502)
A disciple of Ikkyu Sojun (see above), Murato Shuko is considered to be the father of the early Japanese tea ceremony, which is also known as the Way of Tea (see page 12).

Takeno Joo (1502–1555)
The teacher of Sen no Rikyū (see below), Taken Joo was an advocate of Zen simplicity and humility.

Sen no Rikyū (1522–1591)
Sen no Rikyū is credited with developing the details of the Cha-no-yu, or Japanese tea ceremony (see page 12), that are still key today. Rikyu was the tea master for Oda Nobunaga, a Japanese warrior chieftain, and introduced the concept of the slow-paced tea ceremony, making it part of every tough feudal negotiation.

the centuries, in particular towards the end of the 16th century. At this time, having your very own tea master (see page 9) to make your matcha at home was seen as the norm amongst the Japanese elite.

TEA GROWING IN JAPAN OVER THE CENTURIES

Ancient records suggest that the very first batch of tea seeds were planted in Japan in around 805 by two monks, Saicho and Kukai. Following the method they had seen on a trip to China, they pressed the leaves into bricks, and scrapings from the bricks were then put into hot water. The emperor Saga fell in love with tea and encouraged the propagation of tea in Japan, but it wasn't until Eisai (see page 8) promoted matcha in Japan, and brought tea to his friend, the priest Myoe, in Kyoto, that production really took off.

In the 1190s Myoe took matcha plants to many locations including Uji, south-east of Kyoto, where tea cultivation really flourished. This region is climatically suited to tea production with limited frost and a mild but constant wind, and is renowned today for the excellent quality of teas produced there.

Tea producers began to develop and enhance their production techniques in order to optimize the growing, shading and grinding of the very best matcha. It is thought that the shading of the bushes (known as Tana, see page 26) was introduced in the 16th century.

In 1738 Soen Nagatani established the 'Uji green tea processing method'. This is a standard production method that is still used throughout Japan today. His idea was to steam the tea leaves to stop the fermentation process – this method is now called Sencha (see page 24). The Uji method/Sencha gives a fresh, green taste to the leaves. This development was key to tea growing in Japan, making the Japanese green tea unique

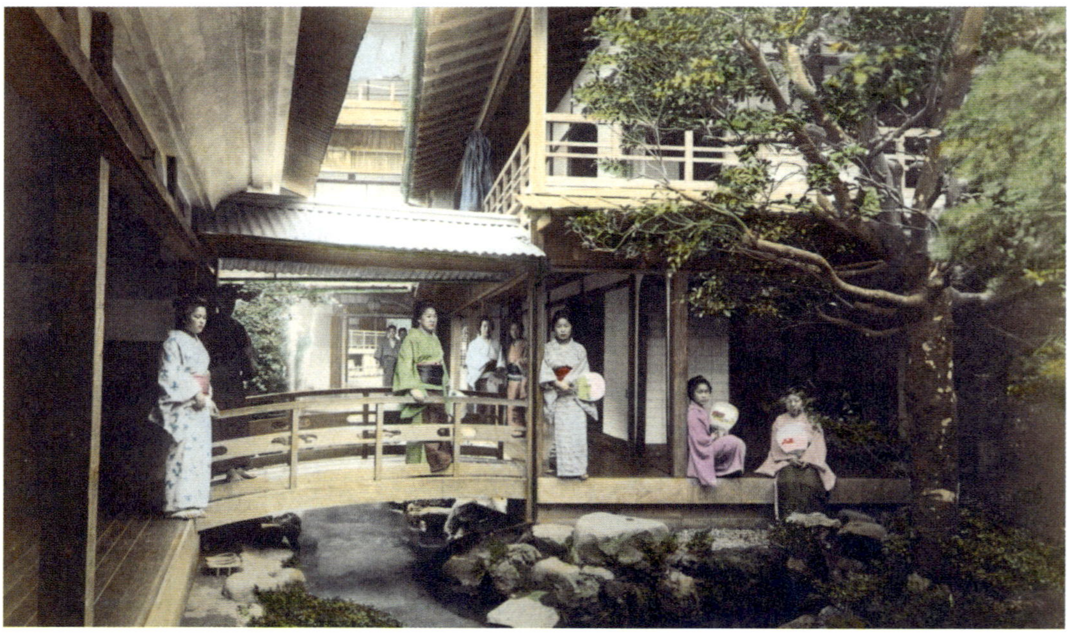

Above Japanese women in traditional clothes inside a tea house, Tonosawa, Japan, c.1880.

and different to the pan-fired or roasted green teas of China. The matcha process includes a gentle steam after the leaves have been picked to retain freshness.

Matcha production has been continually refined over the years and there are now very different qualities of matcha available (see page 28). The number of matcha producers has increased and the standards can vary dramatically between producers.

MATCHA IN THE 21ST CENTURY

Matcha was one of Japan's best-kept secrets, but it is now increasingly consumed around the world. Matcha is a key component of the Japanese tea ceremony (see page 12), where ceremonial-grade matcha is used. Matcha is also widely consumed as a beverage in Japan, and there are several different grades of matcha for drinking (see also page 24).

In addition, the demand for 'ingredient' grade matcha has increased in recent years as matcha began to be used in both sweet and savoury foods. In the last ten years matcha has found its way into some very mainstream products – from ice cream and KitKats to bread and Oreos.

MATCHA HISTORY AT A GLANCE

8TH CENTURY

Green tea made from dried tea bricks drunk widely in China.

960–1129

Chinese Song Dynasty. Steaming and grinding of tea to make a fine powder became popular.

1103

Monastic 'Chanyuan Qinggi' written, describing the etiquette for tea ceremonies in China.

1191

Myoan Eisai, a Japanese monk and founder of Zen Buddhism, brought tea seeds from China, and cultivation and production of matcha started in Japan.

1336–1573

Japanese Muromachi period. Matcha became popular with the Japanese Samurai warrior class.

1522

Sen no Rikyū born. He became a great tea master and formalized the rituals of the Japanese tea ceremony or Cha-no-yu.

16TH CENTURY ONWARDS

Matcha and the tea ceremony firmly established in Japanese cultural life.

21ST CENTURY

Matcha growing in popularity around the world, and is found in everything from cupcakes and croissants to salads and milkshakes.

THE TEA CEREMONY

The Japanese tea ceremony, also called the Way of Tea, focuses on the preparation and serving of matcha in the presence of guests. Although this highly stylized ceremony varies depending on factors such as the season and those participating, it is known worldwide as being a very respectful and peaceful experience.

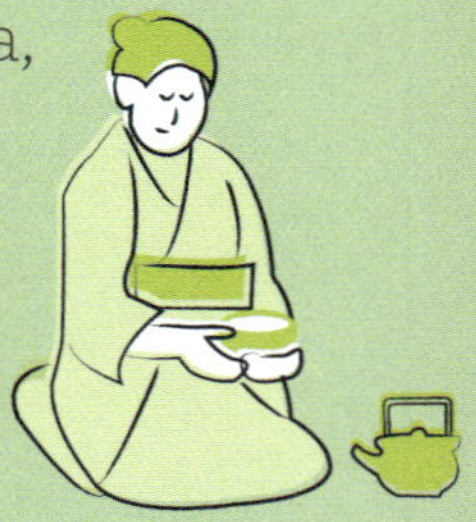

In Japanese the tea ceremony is known as Cha-no-yu (also referred to as Chado or Sado), which roughly translates as 'hot water for tea'. That sounds so simple, doesn't it? Thankfully, from a tea lover's perspective, the tea ceremony is anything but simple. Here is a simple guide to the purpose and practice of the tea ceremony.

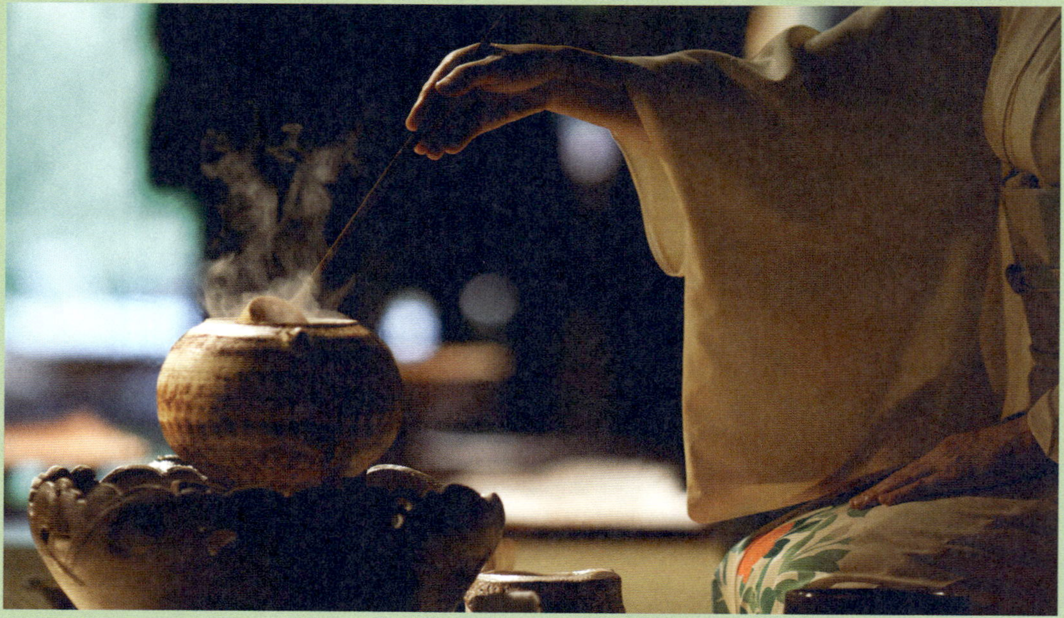

The Four Main Principles of Cha-no-yu

The guiding principles of Cha-no-yu as expressed by Sen no Rikyū (tea master) are:

Wa Complete harmony between guests, hosts and surroundings. This starts from the moment you step into the tea garden.

Kei Profound respect for all, regardless of rank or status. The respect is shown by the kneeling and bowing movements present throughout the ceremony.

Sei To cleanse oneself and be of pure heart and mind. The tea house is supposed to be a refreshing space, the equivalent of a yoga studio!

Jaku Inner peace that you can only discover from obtaining the first three principles of Wa, Kei and Sei.

In addition to these principles, the essence of Cha-no-yu is summed up in ichi-go ichi-e (pronounced eecheego eechee-eh), which literally means 'one time, one meeting'. The participants should be conscious that each tea gathering is a unique occasion so sincerity is key.

Over the centuries the Japanese have perfected the art of tea drinking and preparation. The ritual ceremony is a magical, slow process where the tea is central to a series of precise movements. The enjoyment is supposed to be in two parts: enjoyment of the slow, calm and relaxing steps to make the tea; and enjoyment of the tea itself.

The tea ceremony was fully developed by the 16th century, with professional tea masters such as Sen no Rikyū (see page 9), developing the intricate details that make up the rituals of the ceremony. Every factor is important, from the type of tea, to the ceramics, fashion, painting, flowers, architecture and even the gardens around the tea house. These rituals, surroundings and equipment remain today in Cha-no-yu.

Monks and members of high society traditionally led the tea ceremony (as tea masters), but over time, women became increasingly involved in the ceremony, and today women far outnumber men in the practice of Cha-no-yu.

Left Tea master preparing matcha: taking water with a bamboo ladle (hishaku) from an iron pot (known as a kama or chanoyugama).

WHAT THE TEA CEREMONY INVOLVES

The Japanese tea ceremony is centred on the preparation and serving of matcha in the presence of guests, and a full-length ceremony can last about four hours. Each act involved is designed to focus the senses on the task at hand, and distractions are kept to a minimum.

Each ceremony is unique and will differ depending upon those participating, the time of day, the season and the actual room where it is taking place. That said, the basic procedure for the preparation of the tea always follows certain time-honoured steps (see opposite), and uses key ceremonial utensils (see page 16).

Traditionally the tea ceremony takes place in a room adorned with simple artworks and is accessed by crawling through a low door, thus the participants are immediately required to bow and express humility. The tea master leading the ceremony will have spent years perfecting these ceremonial rituals.

Traditional tatami mats are placed on the floor, and the room is surrounded by Shoji screens, which are window frames filled with paper, shielding the view out so there are no distractions, while allowing light in. Ideally a tea house will be surrounded by a small garden.

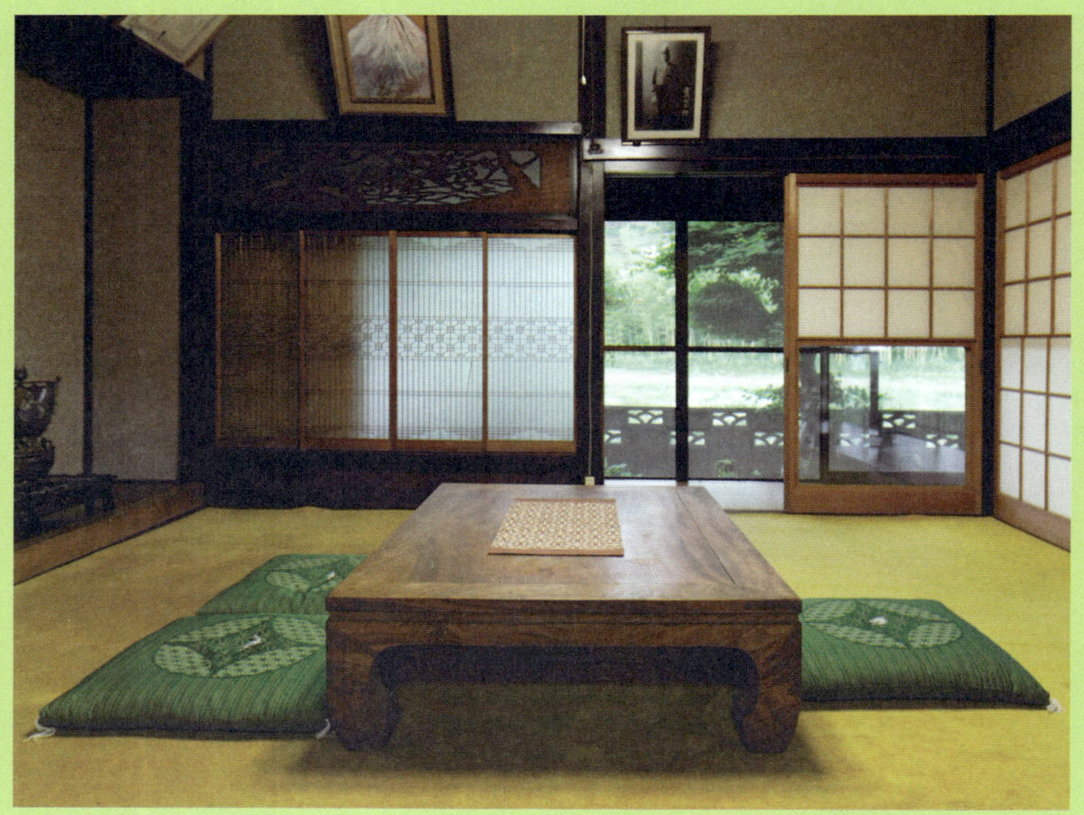

Interior of a traditional Japanese countryside tea house. Tea houses vary in style and size, but simplicity is key.

THE CEREMONY

1 *The guest is greeted by the host with a bow at the entrance gate. The entrance may well be low so the bow is forced.*

2 *The guest washes their hands in a stone wash-basin and they remove their shoes before entering the tea house. This last bit is common practice in all Japanese homes and traditional buildings.*

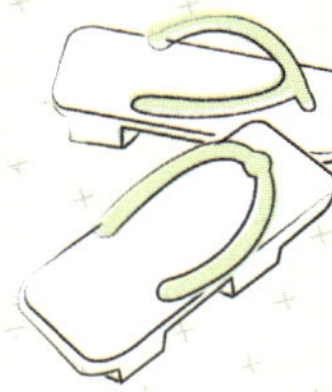

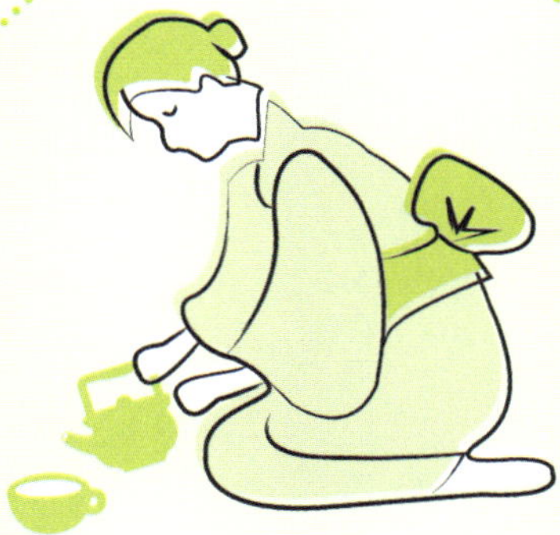

3 *The tea urn, scoop and bowl are wiped down in a symbolic gesture of purification of the utensils.*

4 *Using the scoop, the host transfers the matcha into the bowl and then adds hot water from a kettle using a bamboo ladle. The mixture is then mixed with a bamboo whisk.*

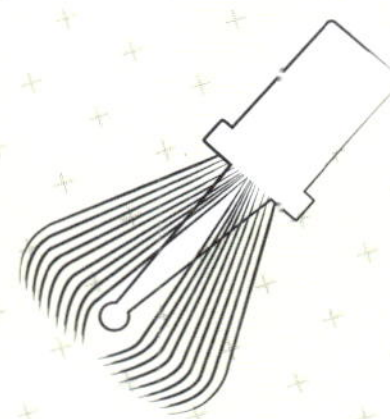

5 *The guest is then offered the freshly made matcha tea and it is placed in front of them. The guest should graciously thank their host with a slight bow of the head.*

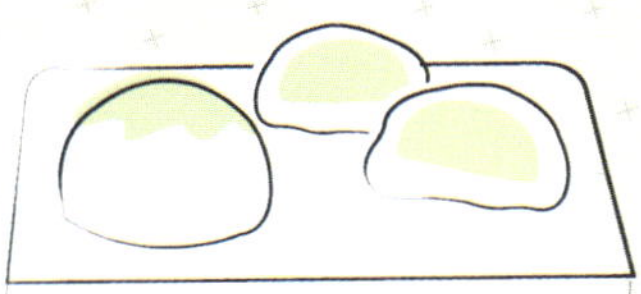

6 *The bowl should be placed in the left hand and guided to the lips with the right. If there is more than one guest, then the first guest wipes the area he/she has just drunk from and passes the bowl to the next guest, who will drink from the same place as the first guest; this gesture is supposed to symbolize the bonding of all those taking part.*

7 *At a full-length ceremony a small meal will be served, however in shorter versions a sweet treat will be offered at the start.*

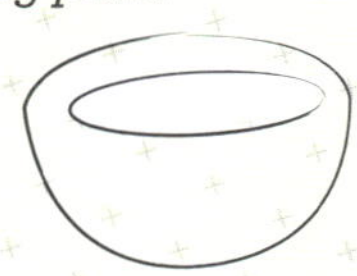

TEA CEREMONY TOOLS

Many utensils are used during the tea ceremony. Collectively they are called 'dogu'. The top three must-haves are the chasen (bamboo whisk), chashaku (tea scoop) and chawan (tea bowl).

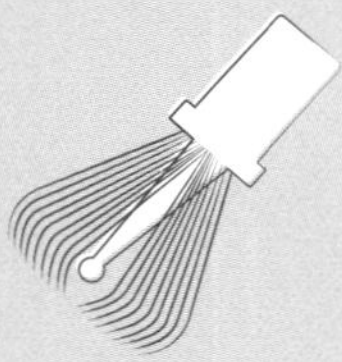

CHASEN *(bamboo whisk): This is the vital element for making matcha. The whisk is carved from a single piece of bamboo and comes with a varying number of prongs. Outside the beautiful world of the tea ceremony we recommend using a speedy milk frother (sacrilege!), however, inside the tea house nothing but this bamboo whisk will do.*

CHASHAKU *(tea scoop): Usually carved from bamboo, the chashaku tea scoop is used to stylishly transfer the matcha from its container to the bowl. It takes a little bit of practice as we are far too accustomed to using a spoon!*

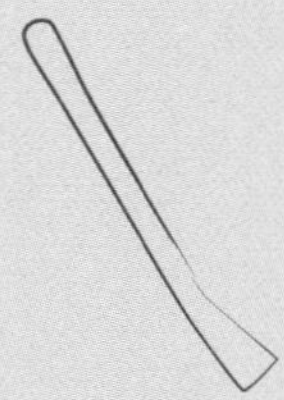

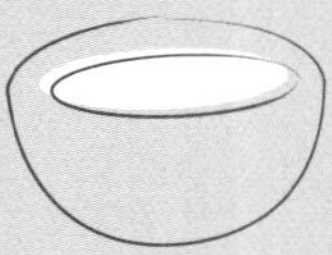

CHAWAN *(tea bowl): In the same way that we have a favourite cup to drink from, the tea master will have a favourite bowl. Some may be ancient and works of great art, hand thrown or heavily decorated, others may be smaller, plainer and just a little cheaper. Interestingly, in summer shallower bowls are used so the matcha chills more quickly. In winter, deep, high-sided bowls are used to keep the tea warm for longer.*

The list of equipment for the tea ceremony is never-ending; if you are a real professional here are some other utensils you may want to use:

Chabako *(storage box for utensils): A solid box containing a set of utensils. A travelling tea master will take his own kit with him.*

Chaki *(pot): The essential pot, used to hold the matcha tea during the ceremony.*

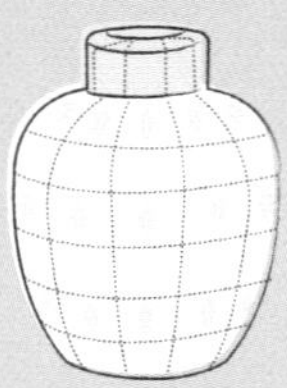

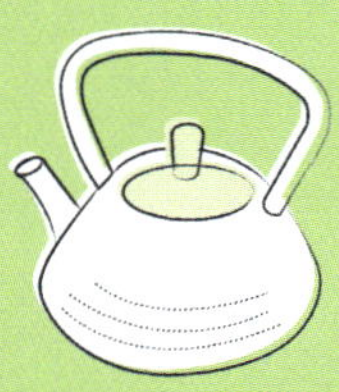

Kama/Chanoyugama *(iron pot): A traditional iron pot used to heat the water for the tea ceremony – a kettle no less.*

Dora *(copper gong): The host gives this a big bang when they are ready for the guests.*

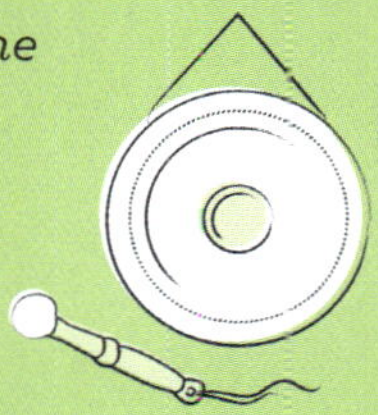

Hachi *(bowl for food/sweets): The special bowl used to present the 'sweet treat' that accompanies the matcha.*

Tenmoku *(tea bowl): A unique tea bowl with narrow feet.*

Kuromoji *(chopsticks): These wooden chopsticks are used to eat the sweet treats. No fingers here!*

Neriko *(incense): A lovely blended incense, which is burnt during the ceremony.*

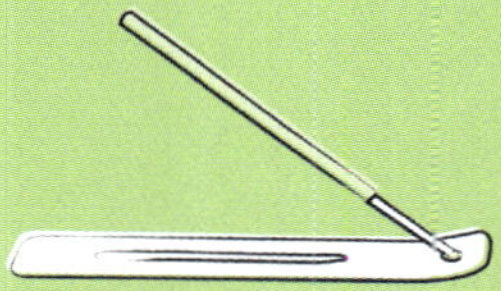

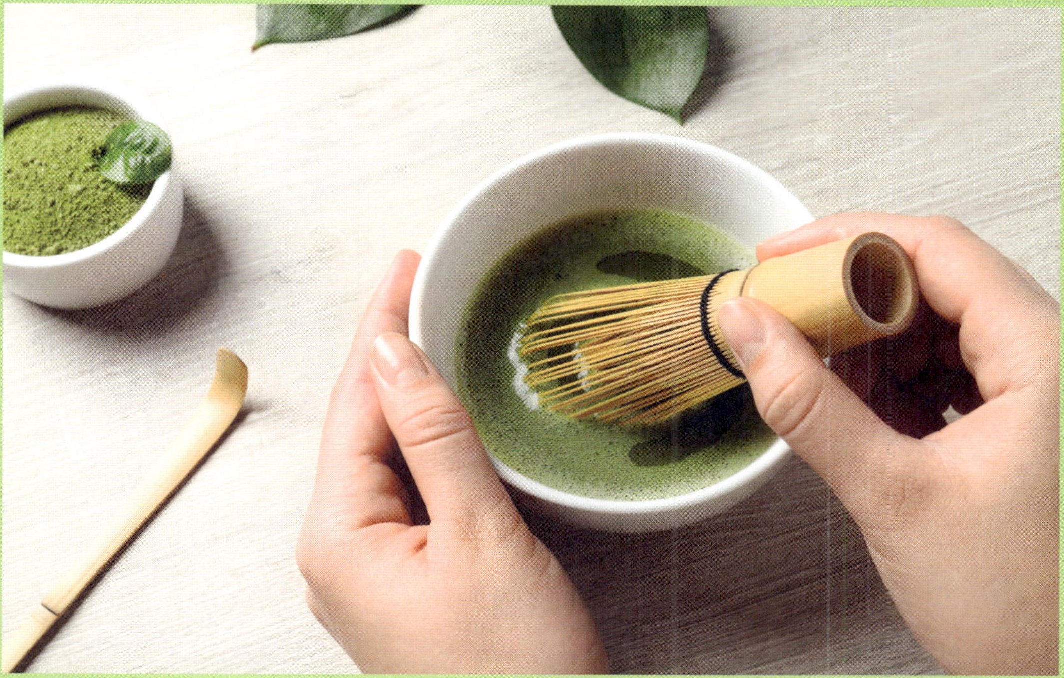

THE DOS AND DON'TS OF THE TEA CEREMONY...

Tourists are often keen to experience a traditional Japanese tea ceremony, and for a fee many places offer this service with an expert or 'host' to guide them through the process (see page 48). If experiencing the ceremony, there are a number of things to remember.

1. First, remove your shoes.

2. If you are game, a kimono will look the part and be respected; if not, 'sensible' Western clothes are acceptable.

3. Enter the room on your knees. Traditionally there is a low door so you have no option other than to shuffle in on your knees.

4. Use only closed fists to balance yourself as you shuffle forward, avoiding the middle of the tatami mats.

5. Know your place! If you find yourself at a tea ceremony you need to know if you are the guest of honour (Shokyaku) or the second in line (Jikyaki). If you are neither of these, you are the Kyaku (a regular guest, don't feel bad!). The Shokyaku will be the first to have the matcha and will pass the bowl to the left, turning and wiping the bowl as it goes down the line.

6. The Shokyaku is the person who thanks the host. The other guests should sit politely and observe the beauty of the room.

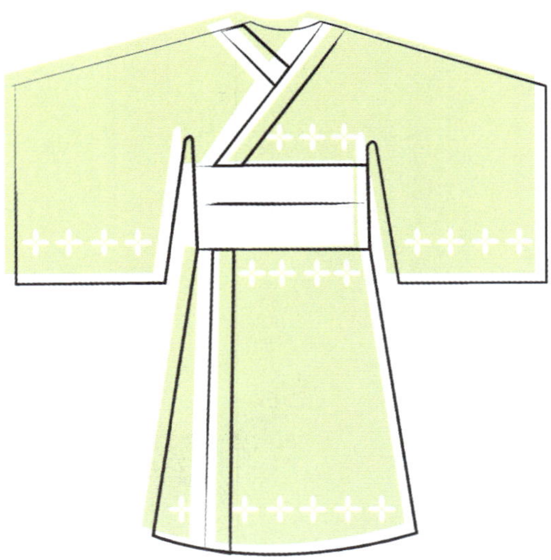

SEASONAL CEREMONIES

Not all ceremonies are the same . . . these are the main seasonal ceremonies.

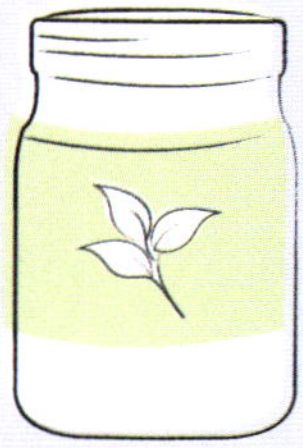

*In **November** there is a ceremony to celebrate the breaking of the seal on a new jar of tea (*Kuchikiri-no-chaji*). This is the first time the tea leaves harvested in the spring will be drunk. The start of the winter season is a great cause for celebration!*

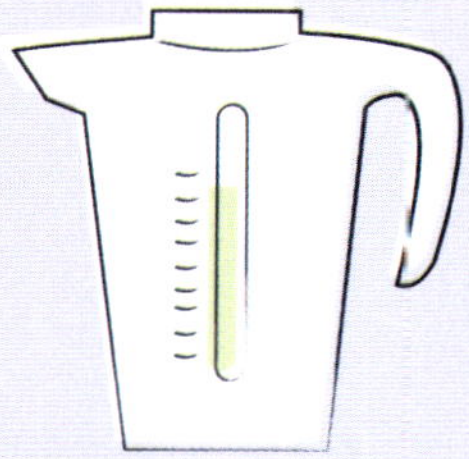

*Held in **January**, the first ceremony of the year is the* Hatsugama, *commonly known as the first boiling of the kettle. This is the fancy pants ceremony, where all the best utensils and sweet treats come out.*

*During the **winter season** there is the dawn tea ceremony (*Akatsuki-no-chaji*), and the dusk ceremony (*Yuuzari-no-chaji*) – these are magical, cold, candlelit ceremonies where you can enjoy sipping tea while watching the sun rise or set.*

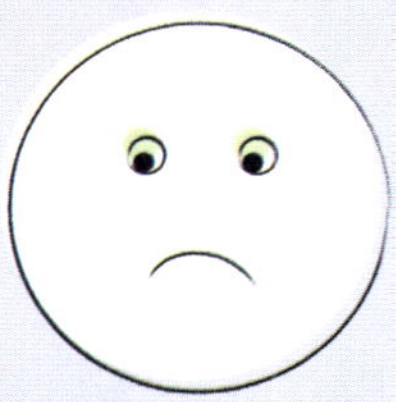

*The end of the tea supply is marked, in **October**, with the* Nagori-no-Chaji *ceremony. This is a sombre event, where the guests display sad faces because of the empty tea jar.*

The production of matcha

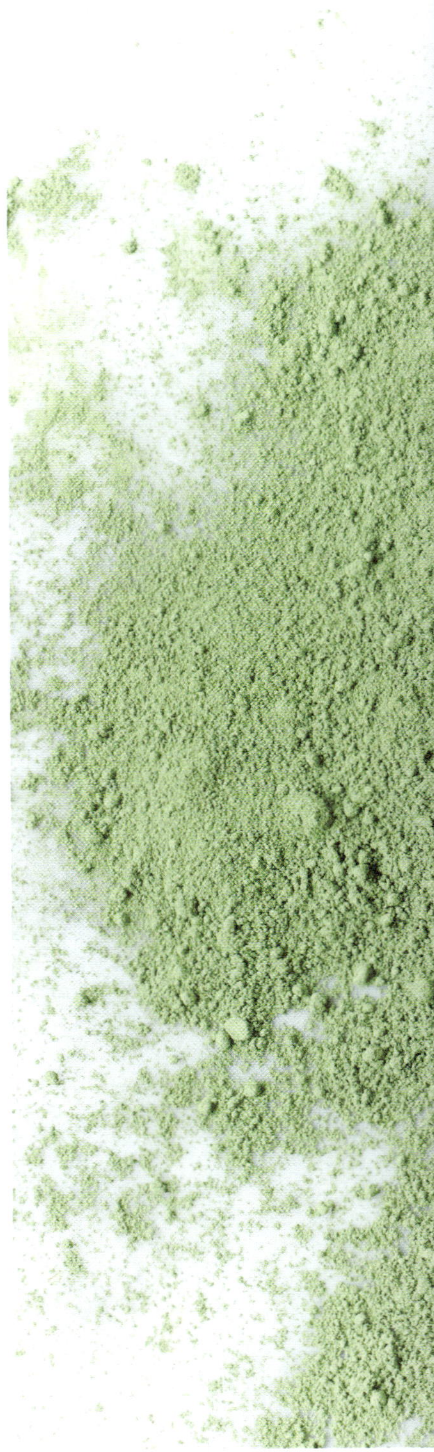

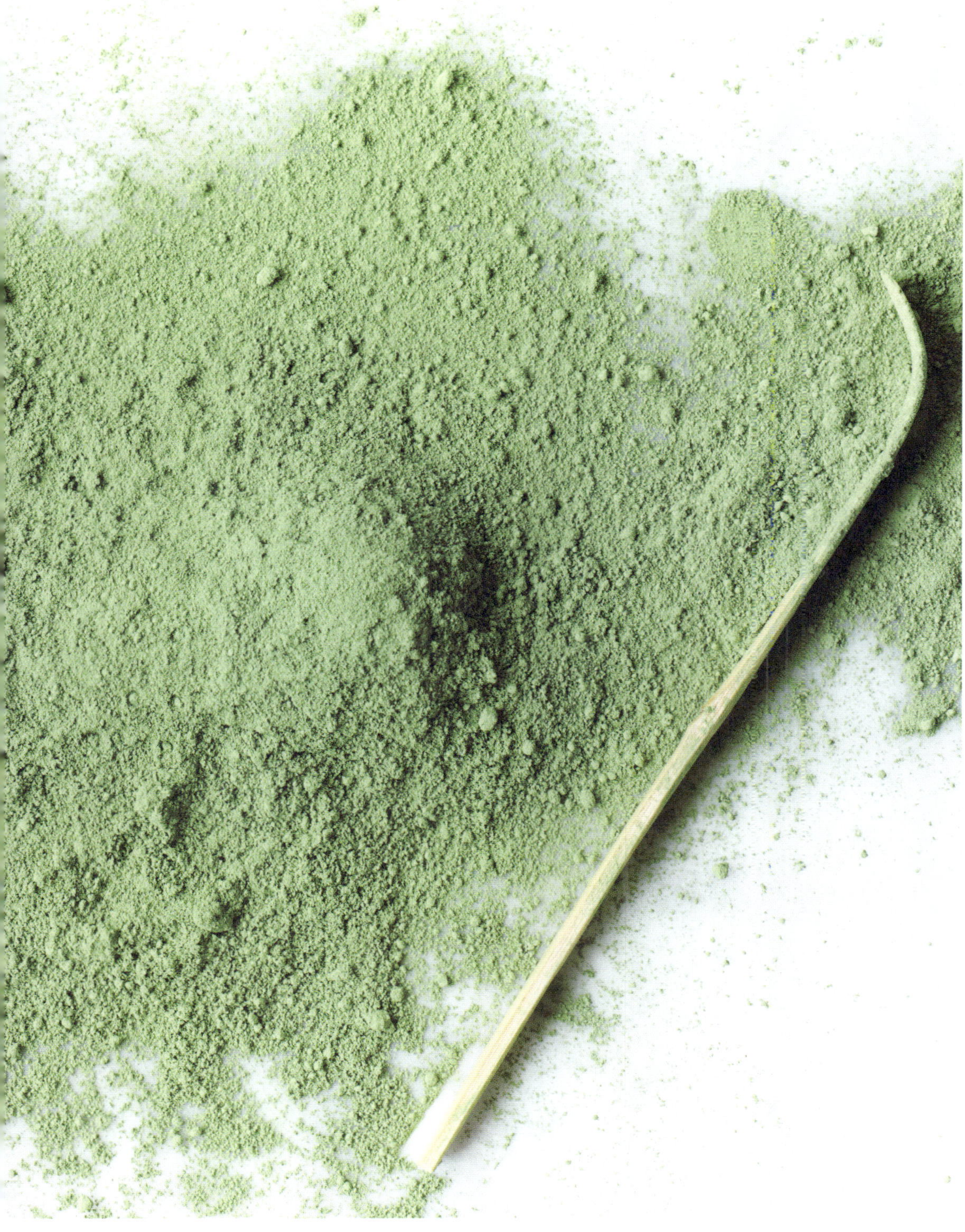

All about tea

Matcha – like all tea – comes from the leaves of the tea plant, *Camellia sinensis*. This subtropical evergreen plant is related to the camellia, a decorative plant grown in gardens. There are two main varieties: *Camellia sinensis var. sinensis*, which is traditionally found in China; and *Camellia sinensis var. assamica*, which is traditionally found in Assam, India.

There are numerous types of tea, which vary widely depending on where they are grown and how they are processed. For example, you will only find the very best white tea growing in the Fujian region in China. The brisk, bright, black tea produced in Rwanda is unique to the mountain region of East Africa. The special fermentation process used in Taiwan generates the most unique oolong tea.

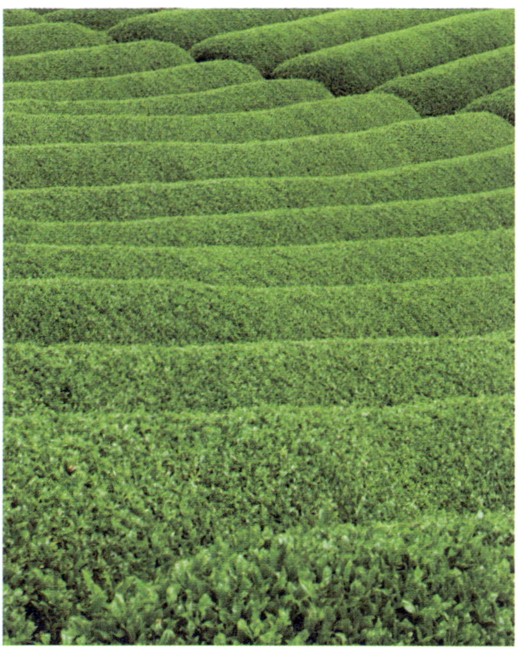

We think it is pretty incredible that one plant can produce so many unique flavours and tastes. The taste variation starts with where the plant is grown – the geographical location, the soil, the altitude and the weather patterns. The defining character is given to the tea by the way the leaves are treated after plucking (picking). This production process changes the final flavour of the tea dramatically.

A good tea is a well-made tea – one that has been looked after and finely crafted at every stage. While the weather patterns can't be controlled, the production stage can be managed very closely. Very generally, tea estates have to choose between making large volumes of 'alright' tea, or a smaller amount of something that is top quality. If they choose the latter they will only pluck the best leaves (the freshest shoots from the top of the bush) and process them very delicately, ensuring that they don't damage the leaf.

Japan is very much the home of genuine, world-class, gold-star matcha, so we will focus mainly on the Japanese tea industry.

Left Rows of fresh green tea bushes growing at a plantation in the Makinohara chabatake tea fields of Shizuoka Prefecture, Japan.

Right Gyokuro tea, a speciality green tea growing under shade in Japan.

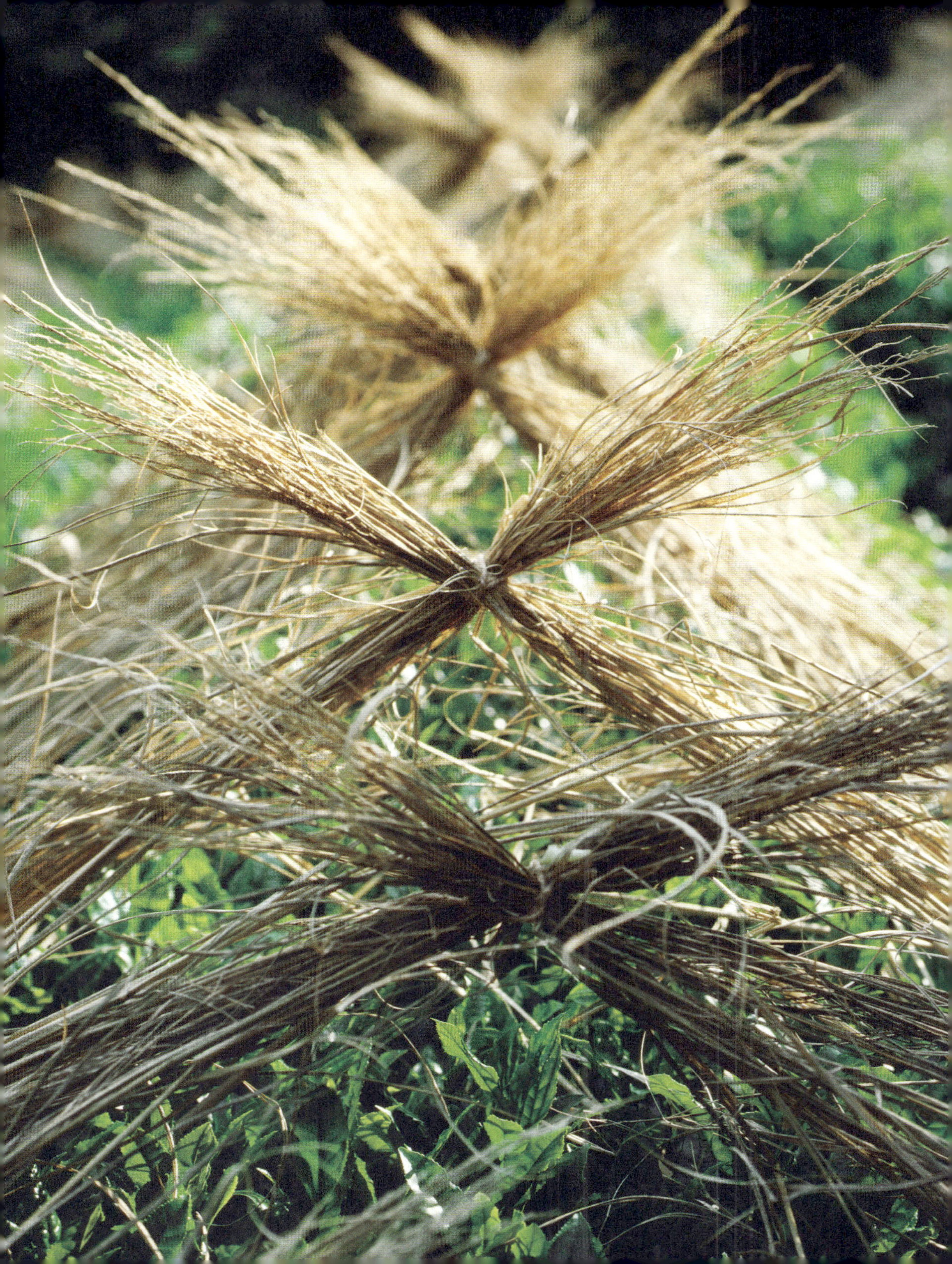

Japanese green teas

The Japanese have taken tea making to another degree with efficient mechanization, which puts them in a different league to other producers. There are only a handful of countries who do not exclusively pluck by hand, but the Japanese have managed to maintain the quality and artisanal approach of tea production despite using machines.

The range of teas produced in Japan is very wide but can be classified into broad categories. Here are six of the top Japanese green teas, if you like, but the list is neverending . . .

1. MATCHA (THE BIG ONE!)

The secret to making matcha from regular green tea leaves is the delicate, complicated, slow production process as shown on pages 26–7. The taste of matcha is unique and its umami flavour (see page 45) can be compared to no other tea produced around the world. Its look is also very different, and although frequently confused with an instant powder, matcha is purely whole leaves ground down to make a super-fine powder.

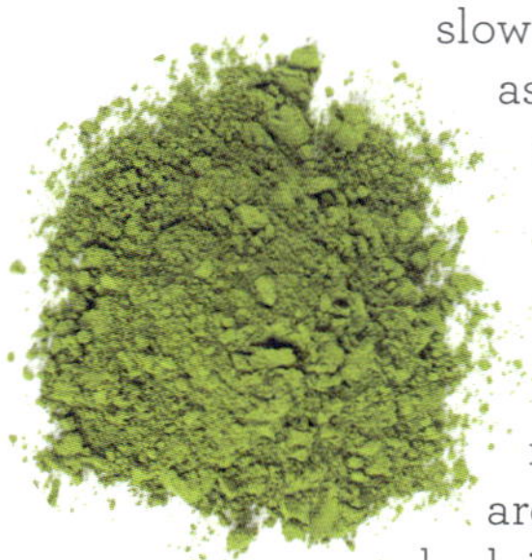

2. SENCHA

Sencha is the most common grade of green tea and makes up about 70 per cent of Japan's total tea production. As explained on page 10, the steaming process was introduced in Uji by Soen Nagatani, and it is the steaming that makes Japanese tea pretty special. The length of time that the tea is steamed for determines its taste: a 20-second blast gives a lighter-coloured cup and a stronger aroma; whereas a longer steam (of up to 160 seconds), which breaks up the leaves more, produces a darker-coloured tea with a stronger flavour.

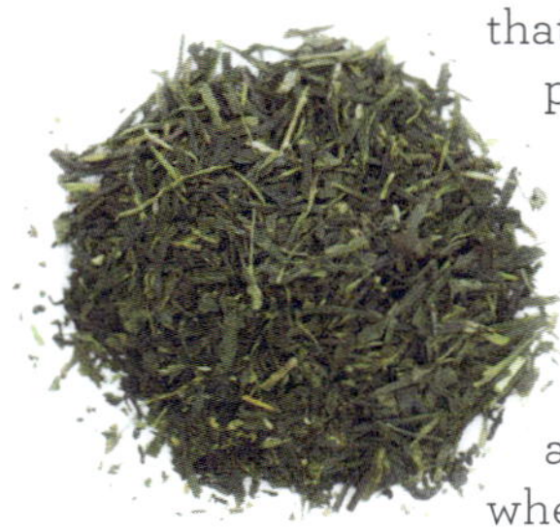

3. GENMAICHA

Genmaicha is made from a sencha green tea base (see above) with toasted and puffed rice added to it. Historically, this tea blend came about as a way of making an expensive commodity (tea) go further. Made for centuries by the poor of Japan trying to save their tea supplies by adding rice, genmaicha

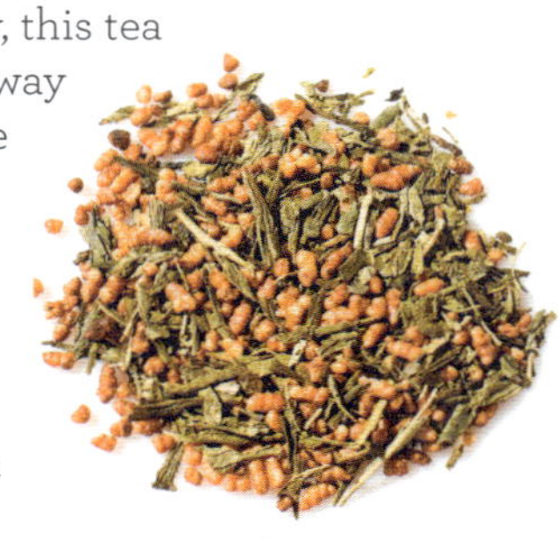

is now one of the most established drinks in Japan. Becoming increasingly popular around the world, this is a teapigs' favourite – we call it 'popcorn tea' as it has hints of popcorn.

4. KUKICHA

Kukicha, also known as bocha and 'twig tea', is a mixture of bright-green sencha leaves (see opposite), or sometimes gyokuro (see right), with yellow leaf stems. Usually, you wouldn't expect good-quality tea made from the stems rather than the buds and leaves of the tea bush, but kukicha is a light, non-astringent and tasty green tea. In addition, as the stems don't contain as much caffeine as the leaves, it's a naturally lower-caffeine drink.

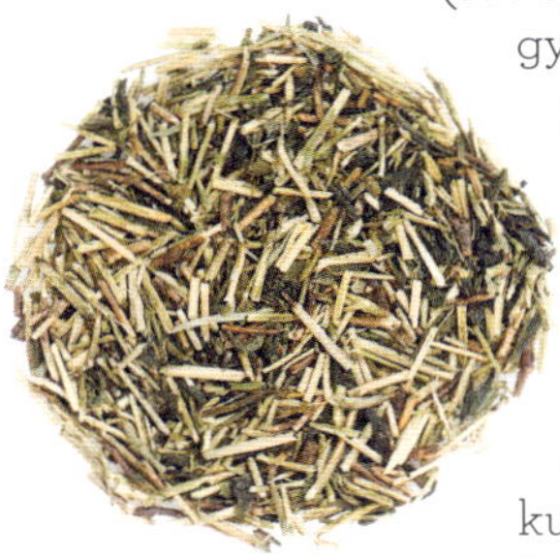

5. HOJICHA

Hojicha is usually made from bancha tea leaves that have been roasted in a porcelain pot over a charcoal fire at a high heat for a few minutes. This distinctive Japanese tea uses the final teas of the harvesting season, and the roasting helps to standardize the flavours. The leaves have a dark brown appearance – not the most appealing to look at but very interesting to taste. The resulting tea is woody and nutty, as well as a distinctive brown rather than green colour.

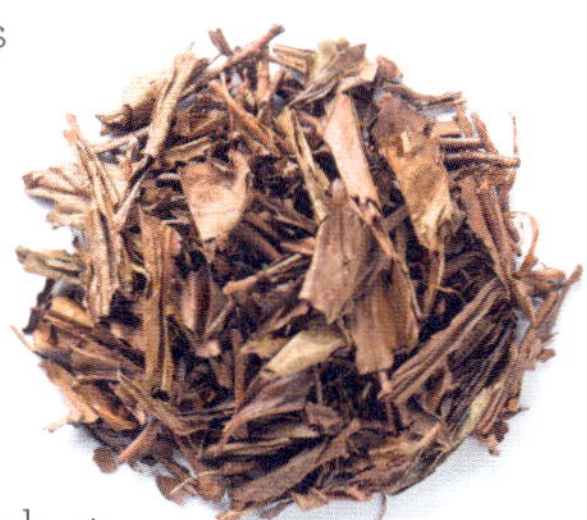

KNOW THE LINGO

Hachiju-hachiya *– 88 nights from the start of spring.*
Tana *– shading over a rack system.*
Jikagise *– less sophisticated shading.*
Aracha *– unrefined tea prior to sorting.*
Tencha *– the base sorted tea prior to grinding.*
Matcha *– superpower green tea – the end result.*

6. GYOKURO

Gyokuro tamahomare (to give it its full name), is one of Japan's most precious teas, revered for its purity and richness of taste. Mainly grown in the area around Kyoto, Japan's ancient capital, gyokuro makes up less than one per cent of Japan's tea production. Produced from just one harvest a year in late May or early June, twenty days before the tea leaves are plucked the tea bushes are covered with a netting. Covering the bushes in this way increases their production of chlorophyll (the pigment that makes leaves bright green) and amino acids. As with matcha (see opposite), the leaves are rich in L-theanine, which gives the tea a lovely sweetness. Gyokuro is also known as 'jade dew', and is one of the most expensive green teas.

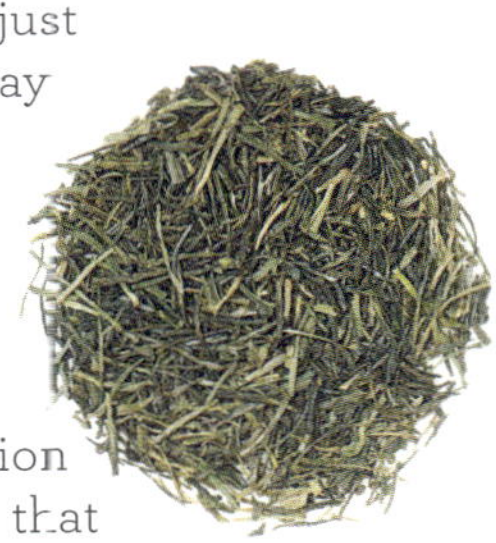

MATCHA PRODUCTION

The secret to making matcha powder, not just ground green tea leaves, is the complicated and delicate growing and production process it undergoes.

Over the winter the tea bushes are cool and dormant. As spring breaks at the end of March to early April, the tea buds begin to shoot. The fields of tea bushes at this stage are almost completely shaded. There are two different ways to shade the leaves – tana and jikagise.

1 The **shading process** stresses out the tea bush. If they could speak, they would be shouting: 'more light, more light!'. The tea bush is unable to photosynthesize and this creates more L-theanine (an amino acid found in tea) and prevents tannins from developing (the tannins give tea its harsh taste). L-theanine also provides the calm energy boost that we look for in matcha and gives a sweet umami taste to the tea (see page 45).

Tana

Tana is used on the large, commercial, top-grade estates and is an elaborate cage that covers the whole field. The cage goes around the edge of the field and over the top of the tea bushes. Netting is spread over the cage with a gap between the roof and the tea bushes to allow growing space. This netting lets in just 10 per cent of the light, yet allows rainfall and moisture to reach the tea bushes.

Jikagise

Jikagise is used by small-scale growers. A large cloth is spread directly over the tea bushes to shade them. This has a similar effect to the tana method but offers less control.

2 *The* **harvesting** *of the tea leaves is done from the 88th day after the start of spring, which is called 'Hachiju-hachiya' in the traditional Japanese calendar. On a modern calendar this usually falls on the first of May.*

3 The **plucked leaves** are taken to the factory to be refined first into what is known as 'aracha' and then into 'tencha'. The leaves are promptly steamed at a very high temperature to stop the fermentation or oxidization process – this keeps the dazzling matcha green colour. The steaming is very short – just 20 seconds. The leaves are then dried slowly to lower the moisture content. At this stage, the leaves are called 'aracha'.

4 The **aracha** (meaning 'rough tea' in Japanese) is then refined further – the stalks, veins and any imperfections are removed. This is done by sieving the leaves, sorting them and using a machine called a colour separator, which pulls out only the perfect bright green leaves for selection.

5 We now have **tencha**. The tencha is then graded, and the graded leaves are ground in a stone mill to make the extremely fine powder we know as matcha.

6 The **stone mill** consists of two granite stones. The stones are engraved with a crisscross pattern, which forces the leaves from the inside of the rotating stones to the outside. The tencha leaves are fed into the gap at the top of the stone mill that joins the stones, which is known as the 'fukumi'. The tencha is sandwiched between the granite stones as they rotate against each other and grind the leaves into tiny particles. The end result is a grain of matcha measuring just 5–10 microns across, which is smaller than a grain of talcum powder! The making of the matcha stone mill is an ancient Japanese art and the grooves in the granite are carved by hand. The miniscule grooves are deeper at the edge of the stone than they are in the middle – this can only be seen with a magnifying glass. Maintaining these traditional granite stones is quite an art, and lifting them is another challenge!

7 The **grinding process** is done in a highly controlled environment. The temperature is cool, consistent and humidity free. The entirely mechanized process is conducted in the dark to keep the leaves bright green and fresh. The grinding process is very time-consuming – to make just one little tin of top-grade matcha takes one whole hour.

The final **matcha** is graded again by an expert tea taster to ensure that the quality is as expected. The ground leaves are then taken to the packing room where, in darkened conditions, the top-grade matcha is vacuum-packed into tins. These tins keep out the light and retain all the freshness of the matcha.

Know your matcha

What is the difference between a green tea powder and matcha? How can you know that you have bought the best matcha, and not a poor imitation? There are a number of things to look out for when buying matcha, including where it's from, its colour and feel, and its cost.

What are the key differences between a green tea powder, which is also marketed in Japan, and a genuine matcha powder?

MATCHA POWDER

Grown in the shade
Bright-green leaf
Steamed
Umami taste (see page 45)
Vibrant colour in cup

GREEN TEA POWDER

Not grown in the shade
Brown/yellow leaf
Pan-fired
Bitter taste
Murky colour in cup

WHAT'S IN A NAME?

There are lots of different types of matcha – ingredient versus premium, ceremonial versus cooking, culinary versus classic. All these descriptions can be very confusing.

Looking at it very simply, some matcha is better for drinking than cooking and some is better suited to cooking. If you are baking matcha croissants or muffins, then ingredient-grade matcha will work well. If you are re-enacting the tea ceremony with fancy guests then you will need the finest, ceremonial-grade matcha. Unfortunately, the words ceremonial and premium are used very freely and there are no labelling restrictions.

QUALITY CHECKING

Telling the quality of matcha from a packet is challenging, but here are a few guidelines:

1. Matcha should always come from Japan, in particular Uji and Nishio (see opposite).
2. Look out for a recognized brand name.
3. Matcha should come in a high-quality airtight container, whether tins or sachets.
4. The packet should have a proper organic certification.

If you have bought a top-quality matcha it should be:

- a bright grass – almost neon – green.
- sweet and not at all bitter.
- smooth to the touch, not grainy.

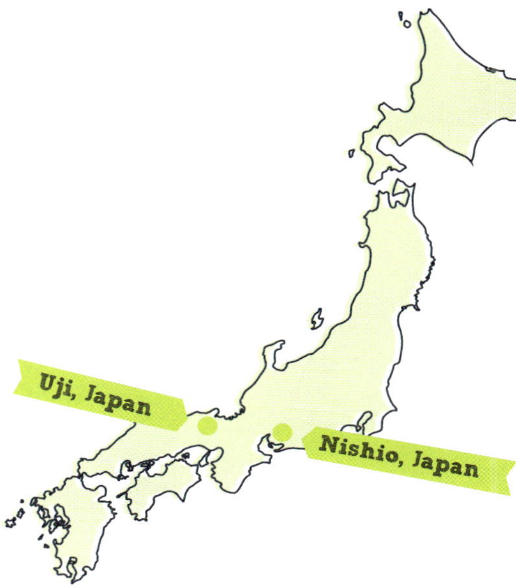

MATCHA PRODUCTION REGIONS

In Japan there are two 'best-in-show' matcha production areas.

1 **Uji** is a small city on the southeastern outskirts of Kyoto and is one of the oldest cultural centres in Japan. This area is famed as being the original birthplace of tea in Japan and is renowned for its high-quality green teas. The region is frost-free due to the mild constant winds and it has perfect growing conditions for matcha production.

2 **Nishio** is a city in the Aichi Prefecture and is the largest producer of matcha. For centuries it has been a major tea-growing region and has an ideal climate for growing matcha, with a fertile soil and mild, wet weather pattern.

Not only is Nishio the largest producer of matcha green tea, it is also the largest producer of unagi freshwater eels (unrelated but interesting!).

MATCHA AROUND THE WORLD

The crucial elements required to produce a great-quality matcha are the growing conditions, the shading and the grinding (see pages 26–7). These have been perfected over the centuries in Japan, where matcha has been so important in the tea ceremony, so we need to look primarily to the Japanese for great matcha.

However, around 15 years ago, China began to produce larger volumes of ground green tea to compete with the Japanese matcha market. A form of 'matcha' is even being produced in Kenya, where it is ground from white tea; and 'red matcha' is being ground from rooibos in South Africa. Although nowadays there is a liberal use of the word 'matcha', we should really be thinking of quality shade-grown green tea from Japan when we see the word 'matcha'.

Matcha producers today

The tea industry can be seen everywhere in the countryside in Uji, in Kyoto Prefecture, and in Nishio, in Aichi Prefecture (see also page 29), which are the two main tea and matcha producing areas in Japan. The land here looks very different to other tea-growing regions worldwide, as their undulating fields are uninterrupted. Here, roads are sandwiched between verdant green tea fields or less-attractive shaded fields in the spring.

THE MATCHA PRODUCERS

The producers in Japan are dominated by one major player, who manufactures 80 per cent of the Japanese matcha in Aichi Prefecture. There are also multiple small tea growers in Japan – from tiny family growers with small plots, to slightly larger commercial growers. These growers sell their freshly picked 'green leaf' to the larger matcha manufacturers, which means that the dominant matcha manufacturers do not exclusively grow all the matcha in Japan.

MATCHA PRODUCTION AS PART OF THE WORLD TEA PRODUCTION

Over six million tonnes of tea are cropped in the world every year. A mere 4,000 tonnes of which are produced as matcha in Japan – that means just 0.07 per cent of all teas produced globally are sold as matcha.

To make most types of tea you need four kilograms of green leaves to make one kilogram of tea. However, to make one kilogram of ground matcha requires more than six kilograms of fresh green leaves – the extra amount is necessary because the veins and stalks are removed as part of the production process (see also page 27). This, along with the complex production process and unreliable weather patterns affecting the harvest yield, inflates the price of matcha, making it justifiably more expensive than regular tea.

Matcha production has increased by nearly three times the quantity grown in 2010, with many tea growers switching to tencha planting. Even though the majority of matcha is still consumed within Japan, domestic and international demand has exploded in the last few years.

THE CHANGING MATCHA INDUSTRY

The matcha industry has changed considerably since the export market became more established. teapigs were the first company to bring matcha to the UK in 2008, and since then the matcha industry in the UK has flourished. Demand has also grown considerably in other European countries and in the USA and China in particular. It is now common to see matcha on the menu in leading cafés and restaurants around the world (see also pages 50–51). This has resulted in an increased demand for fine matcha in Japan and for ingredient-grade matcha for use in matcha-flavoured food and drinks, which is good news for the producers.

Although most matcha is not produced organically, the demand for organic matcha has also increased in recent years.

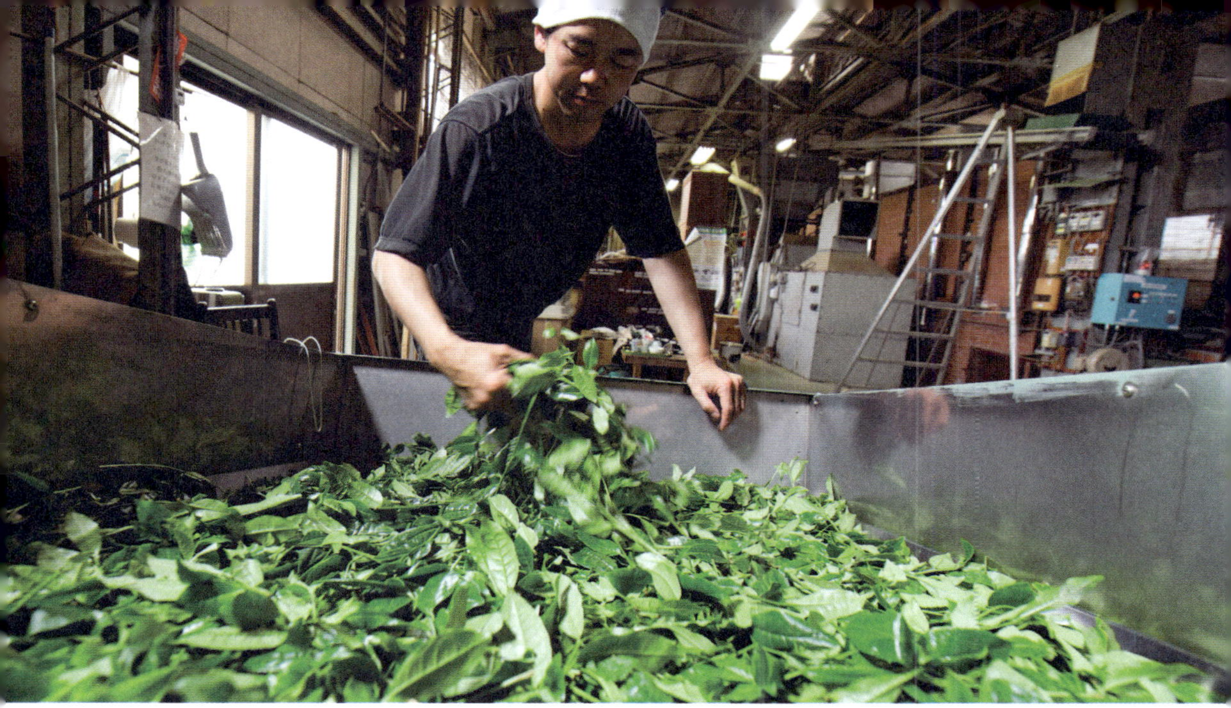

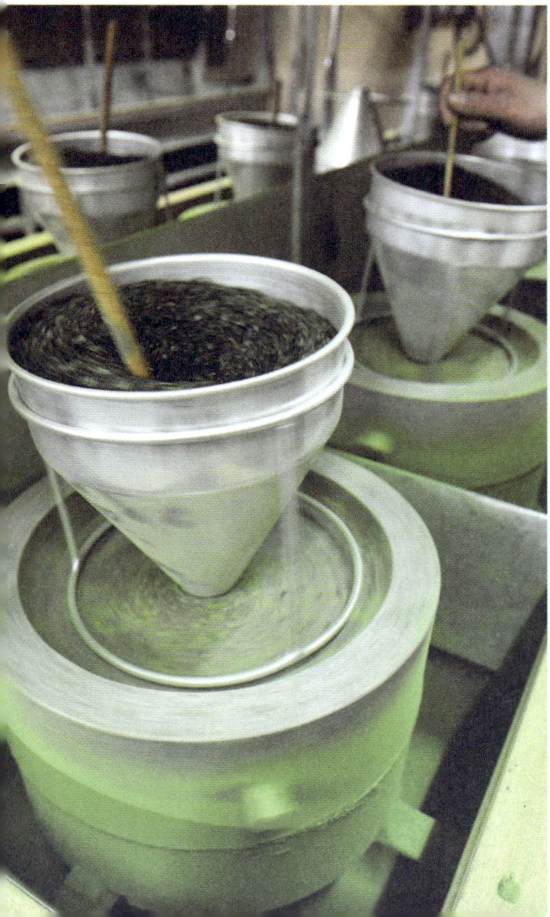

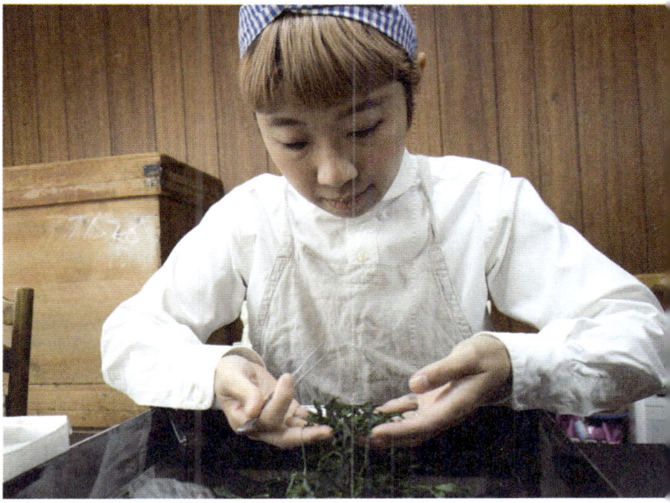

Top Freshly picked tea leaves being steamed.

Bottom left Tencha leaf being ground down on stone grinders to make matcha powder.

Bottom right Sorting the leaves carefully for grading quality.

The health benefits

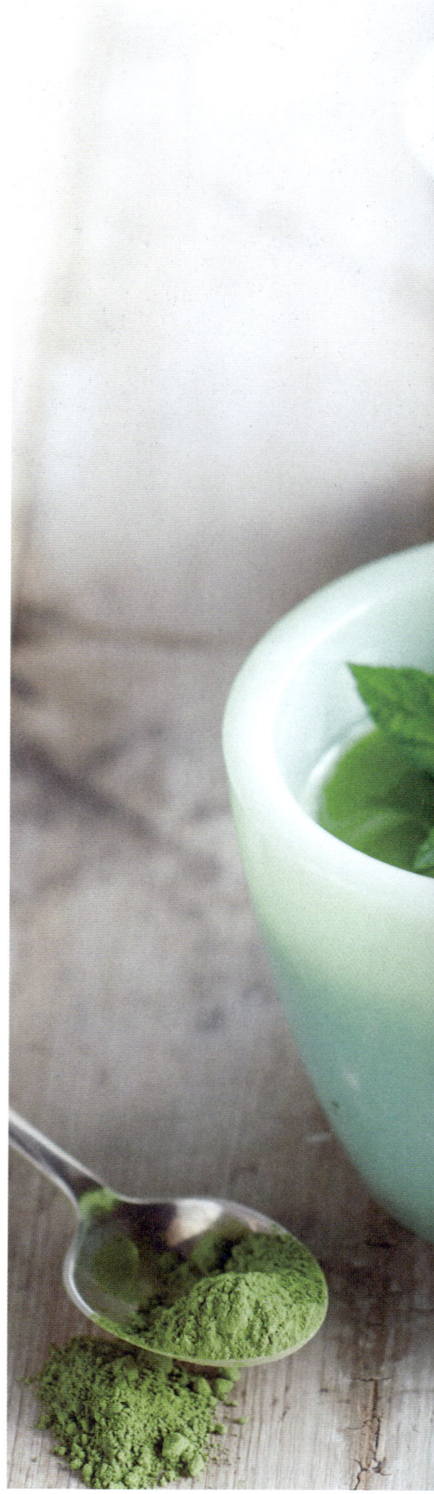

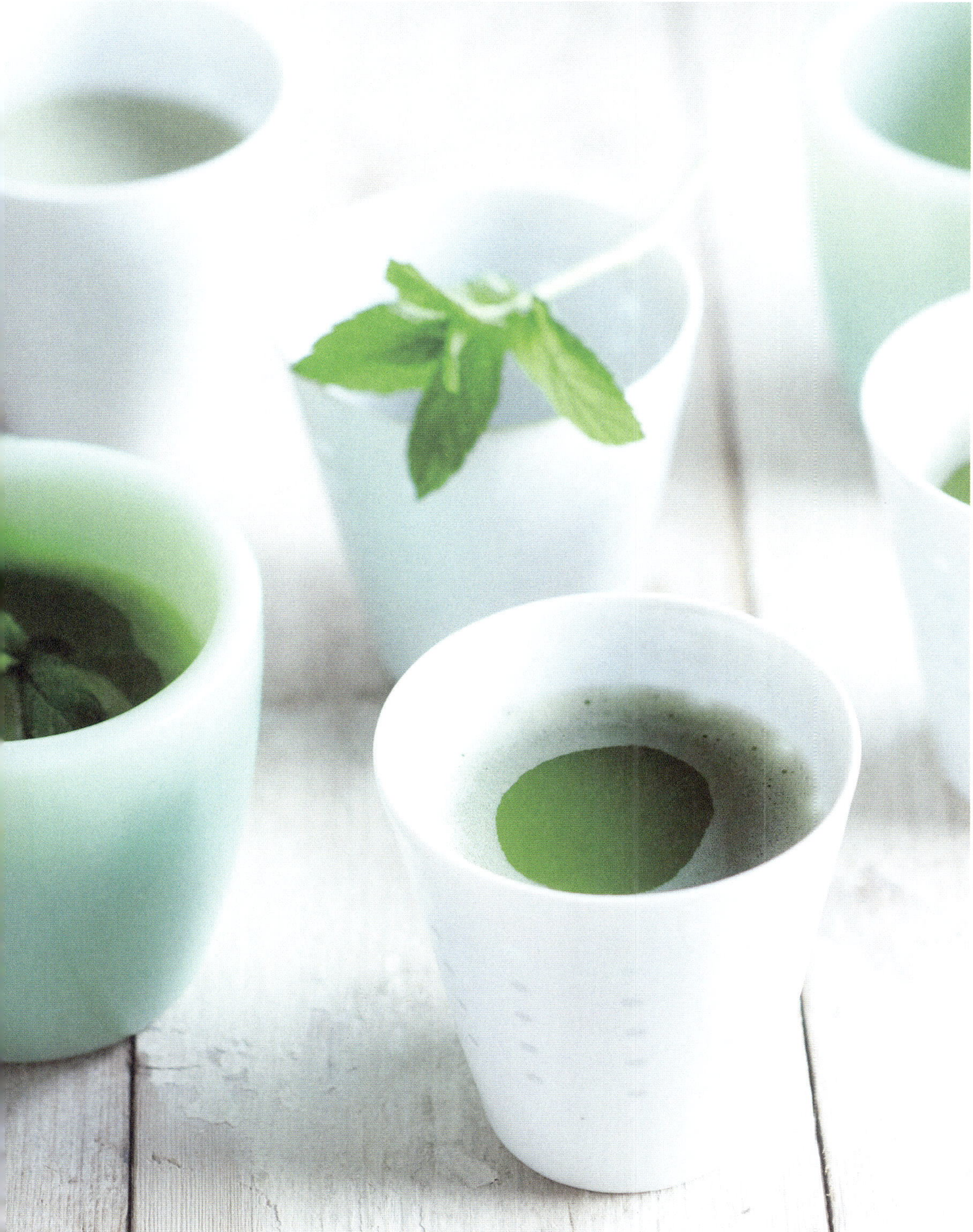

The 'superpower' green tea

We all love a cup of delicious, top-quality green tea. Here we will help you to understand why adding this 'superpower' green tea to your diet will make you feel a little bit more . . . super!

The secret to matcha is obvious when you start to learn more about this superpower drink. There are two main reasons why matcha is so amazing:

1. The way it is grown and produced.
2. The way it is drunk.

1 THE POWER OF SHADE

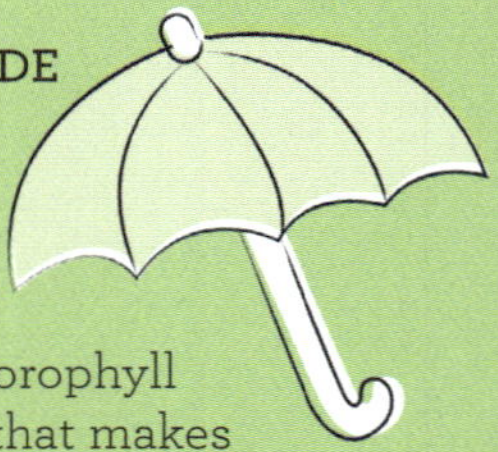

Matcha bushes are grown under lots of shade, which boosts the production of amino acids and the chlorophyll content (that's the stuff that makes the leaves their lovely bright-green colour). The leaves are then hand-picked and all the stems and veins are removed, leaving only the juiciest, most nutrient-rich leaves. The leaves are ground by granite stones to a super fine powder, which is packed immediately to preserve all the nutrients. See The production of matcha, page 20.

'SHADING THE TEA BUSHES BOOSTS THE AMINO ACID AND CHLOROPHYLL CONTENT; WHILE CONSUMING THE WHOLE LEAF MEANS YOU GET EVERY LITTLE BIT OF MATCHA GOODNESS.'

2 A PACKED CUPPA

That brings us to our second secret – the way matcha is drunk. When you drink regular green tea, whether loose tea or in a tea bag, you throw away the leaves after you have let them infuse. This is a bit like boiling spinach, throwing away the spinach and just drinking the water – you will get some of the nutrients, but you're discarding the best bit – the leaves with all the nutrients.

When you drink matcha, you mix the bright-green, nutrient-rich powder into liquid and ingest the entire tea leaf. Every little particle is packed with goodness, so when you knock back your matcha, you're consuming every tiny bit of that lovely green tea.

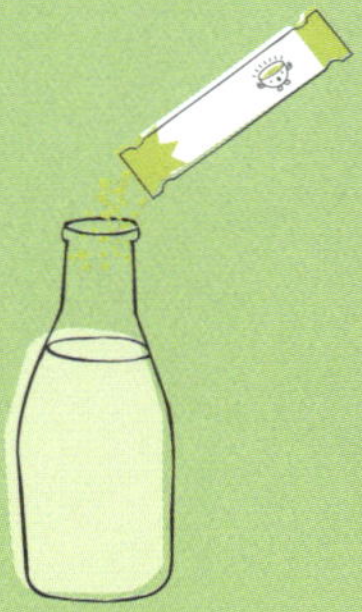

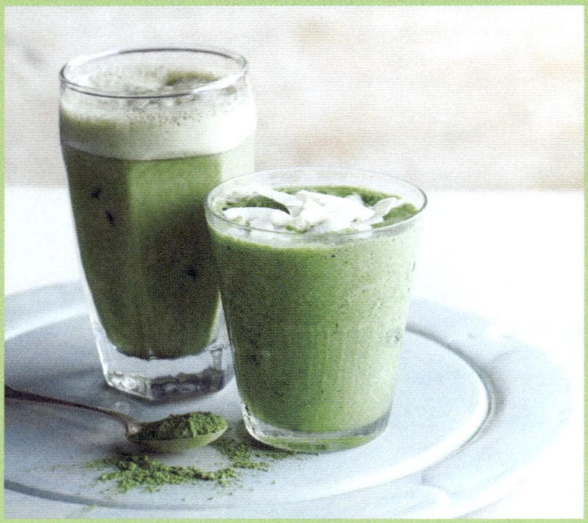

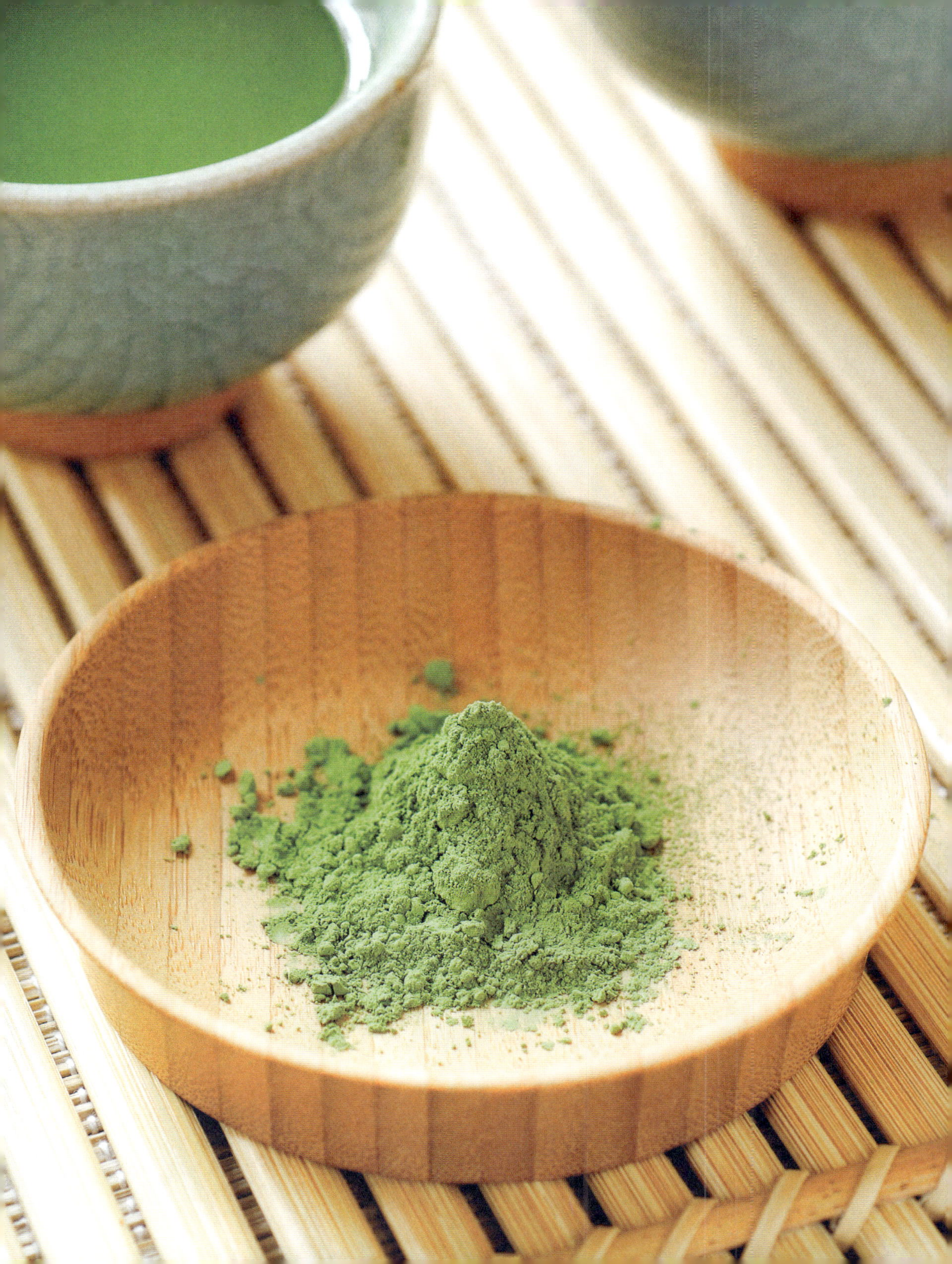

Matcha's health benefits

Why is matcha so good for you? Why does it make you feel great? Why is it a superb alternative to regular green tea? Why should you swap your favourite cup of the black stuff for this bright-green brew?

GREEN TEA FLAVONOIDS

EGCG is big news – not heard of it? Matcha contains high amounts of natural green tea flavonoids known as catechins. EGCG (for those, like us, who cannot pronounce its chemical name), or epigallocatechin gallate in full, is a major catechin. Many of the studies that have investigated the antioxidant power of matcha have focused on how EGCG works within the human body. See also page 38.

WHAT CAN MATCHA DO FOR YOU?

Dazzling skin

Green tea contains polyphenols, and researchers at the University of Alabama have found that consumption of green tea polyphenols can inhibit UV-radiation-induced skin damage [1].

It is well known that the sun's UV rays can damage skin, cause premature ageing and even cause skin cancer. Their study found that these polyphenols can be used to prevent sun-induced skin disorders, helping to keep your skin looking healthy.

Calorie burning

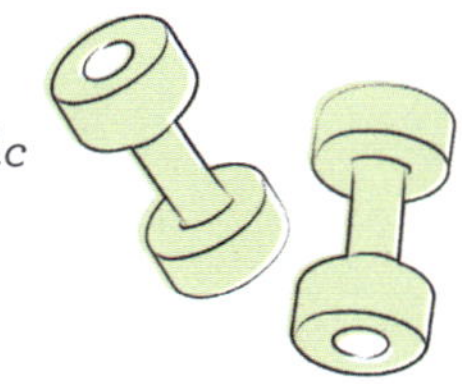

A large number of scientific studies are looking at the effect that green tea may have on the body's thermogenesis (that is, the rate it burns calories) and on its impact upon fat oxidization during exercise *(see also page 39).*

Green tea extract is now used in many slimming supplements.

Matcha is probably the purest and most natural form of green tea extract – and lovely to drink, too.

Energy, concentration and focus

As with all types of green tea, matcha contains caffeine, which is a natural stimulant. Matcha also contains an important amino acid called L-theanine. These two compounds appear to work together to give a slow release of energy, rather than a quick energy boost and then a dip, and many drinkers report that they feel alert and focused for a number of hours after they consume matcha. Much research has been – and continues to be – conducted into how L-theanine may help promote alpha brain waves, which are known to help with concentration *(see also page 41).*

Focus

Matcha is believed to give you a slow release of energy that lasts throughout the day while keeping you calm, alert and focused at the same time. That's why Japanese students drink it when they're cramming for their exams, and it's also why Buddhist monks have always drunk matcha to help them meditate.

Drinking matcha is like drinking 10 cups of regular green tea for its nutrient value – no wonder people consider matcha a superpower green tea.

Extra oomph

Lots of athletes are discovering the benefits of drinking matcha while training. Olympic swimmer, Rebecca Adlington, is a big matcha fan.

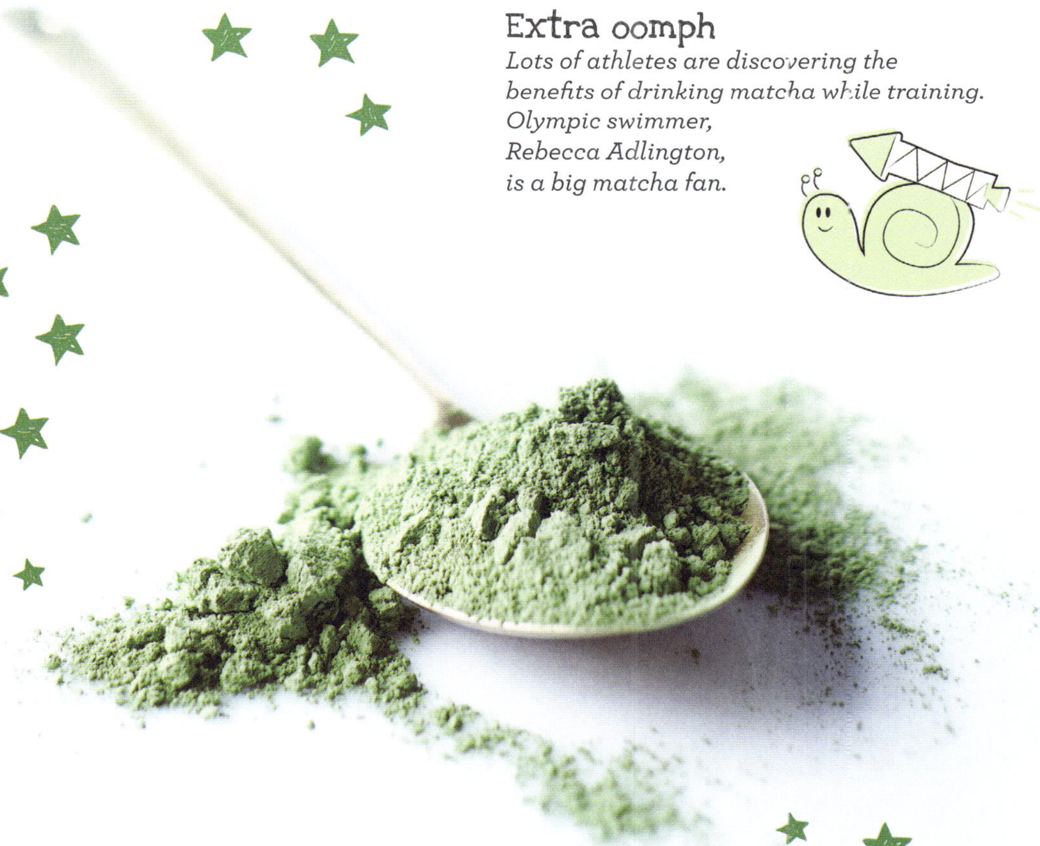

'MATCHA IS AN ALL-NATURAL BEVERAGE THAT HAS BEEN DRUNK FOR CENTURIES FOR ITS AMAZING PROPERTIES.'

The experts' view

Now you know a little about the history, culture and production of matcha, here's some of the science behind why it's so great. Top nutritionists and authors of bestselling book *The Sirtfood Diet*, **Aidan Goggins** and **Glen Matten**, have delved into the varied and notable health benefits of matcha. Experts in the field of health and nutrition, Aidan is a trained pharmacist and nutritionist, while Glen has a master's degree in nutritional medicine.

A little-known fact is that matcha green tea was Europe's original tea. In the early 1600s Dutch traders set up in Japan, where matcha was the tea of choice. Upon its discovery it was sent to Europe where it quickly became very popular. However, changes in supply meant a switch to black tea some 100 years later. But with matcha green tea readily available once more, by going green everyone can again enjoy this delicious beverage and all its health-giving wonder.

The reason tea is believed to be so good for us is primarily down to its rich content of a group of powerful plant nutrients called catechins, and especially a particular one – epigallocatechin gallate (EGCG). (See page 36.) Whereas black tea only contains about 3–10 per cent catechins, green tea boasts a staggering 30–40 per cent, with matcha by far the best green tea catechin source.

In order to truly appreciate matcha, first we need to look at the amazing health benefits of the catechins and EGCG that modern science has unearthed, before looking at what marks matcha out as being the supreme form of green tea.

GREEN TEA CATECHINS AND HEALTH

Cancer

A large and still growing body of laboratory, animal and human research suggests an important role for green tea in cancer prevention. Significant benefits have been observed for green tea consumption, and especially EGCG, for inhibiting cancer growth in the prostate, lung, stomach and breast [1–4].

With benefits for such a broad range of cancers, low toxicity, and the fact it is easy to consume with low risk of side effects, researchers are now looking to green tea as a potential inclusion alongside more conventional cancer medicines.

Heart health

When it comes to matters of the heart, there is much love for green tea.

A 2014 review, which combined the results from 20 trials, found that green tea consumption has significant benefit for lowering blood pressure and cholesterol [5].

But how does that translate to the chances of actually succumbing to heart disease? A large Japanese study of 40,530 adults found those who enjoyed five cups or more of green tea daily had a 26 per cent reduction in death from cardiovascular disease compared to those consuming just one cup a day [6].

Diabetes

There has been considerable interest in the benefits of green tea for diabetes and improving blood sugar control.

In 2013 an analysis of 17 trials put this to the test and found that green tea consumption significantly lowered levels of fasting blood sugar and a measure called HbA1c, which indicates long-term blood sugar levels [7].

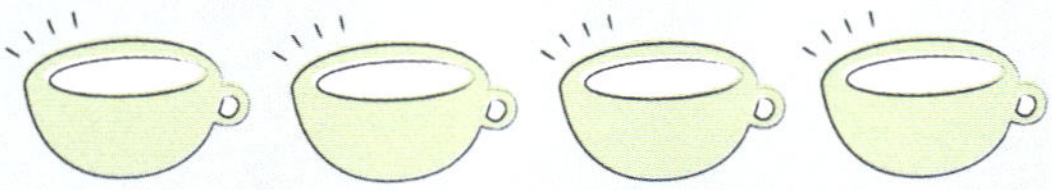

The real-world effect of these benefits are shown when researchers pulled together all relevant studies that have looked at the relationship between tea drinking and diabetes risk. The results of this analysis show that drinking more than 3–4 cups of green tea a day reduces the risk of type 2 diabetes by around 15–20 per cent when compared to non-tea drinkers [8, 9].

Bone health

Green tea is now also emerging as an invaluable food in the battle against osteoporosis. Early stage studies show that catechins enhance bone formation and suppress bone breakdown. Studies from countries around the world, including the UK, link tea consumption as a protective factor against osteoporosis. And one early stage intervention study of 150 post-menopausal women with early stage osteoporosis found that consuming green tea catechins (equivalent of 4–6 cups of green tea a day) for six months reduced bone stress, helped to boost bone formation and improved muscle strength [10].

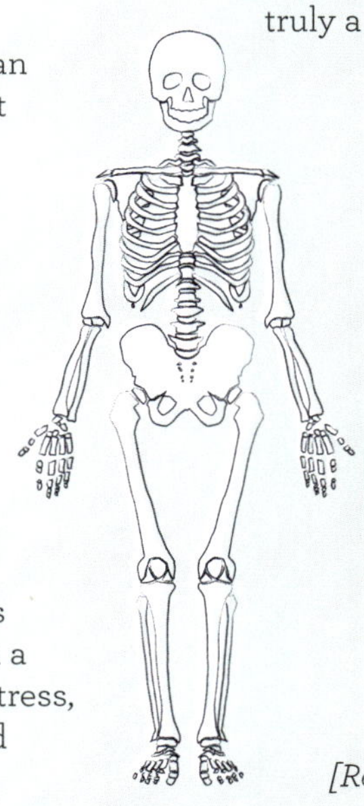

'WE LIKE TO REFER TO MATCHA AS GREEN TEA ON STEROIDS.'

Weight

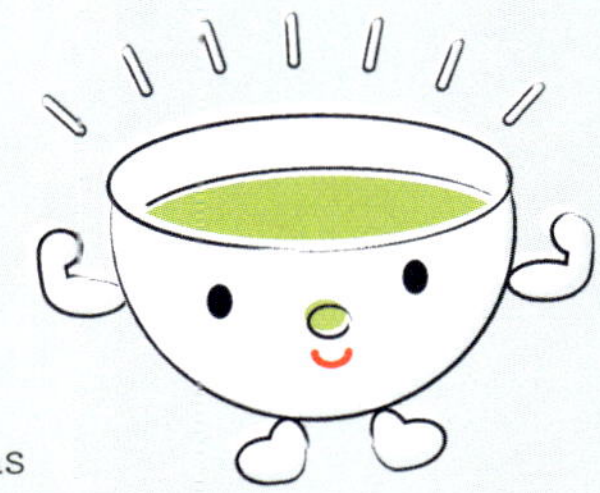

Green tea has received much hype as a weight loss aid, but what's the science?

Green tea catechins exert a thermogenic effect, which means they help drive fat burning in the body, making it a valuable aid in the battle of the bulge. Habitual green tea drinkers have been shown to have a 20 per cent reduction in body fat percentage as well as a favourable reduction in their waist-to-hip ratio [11].

Drinking green tea also shows benefits for maintaining fat loss after people stopped dieting, as well as in enhancing the fat-burning effects from exercise, making it truly a food for improving body shape.

Look out for the 'Nutritionists' logos in the recipe section, as these highlight the super-healthy recipes chosen by Aidan and Glen.

[References given on page 174.]

Green tea as a wonder Sirtfood

As practising clinicians in the field of Nutritional Medicine, Aidan and Glen are well versed when it comes to recommending specific foods for treating specific conditions. However, green tea transcends this, so broad are its health benefits. Here they look at matcha's advantages.

It seems that there are very few people who would not benefit from drinking green tea regularly, which begs the question – how can one food do so much?

It's all down to the fact that green tea, and especially matcha, is one of a newly discovered group of wonder foods called Sirtfoods. These foods contain especially high levels of special nutrients that switch on a master group of genes that exist in all of us, called sirtuins.

When our sirtuins are turned on they activate a recycling process in our cells that clears out the cellular debris, which accumulates over time causing ill health and loss of vitality. To fuel this recycling process the body uses our fat cells. The result of activating our sirtuin genes means we increase our sense of wellbeing, we boost our resistance to disease and we burn significant amounts of fat in the process. Activating sirtuins has been shown to be a key factor in preventing the many chronic diseases that afflict us, explaining why green tea has such wide-ranging benefits in these conditions.

Until now, the benefits of foods have been judged on the basis of their content of vitamins, minerals, antioxidants and other nutrients that nourish the body. The discovery of sirtfoods has changed all this.

Sirtuins are not turned on through nourishment; in fact it is the opposite. They are only turned on when the cells in our body are stressed. Indeed, the reason green tea is so good for us is that the catechins (especially EGCG) act like weak toxins that actually stress the cells in our body.

At first thought, the idea that stress or toxins could be really good for us might seem really odd, but bear with us.

What we are talking about is a controlled, physiological stress, caused by these natural plant compounds. This low-level 'stress' switches on our sirtuin genes, which ramp up the efficiency of our cells, causing them to adapt to the stress and become fitter and healthier and more hardy against future stresses. By repeated exposure to this low-level stress our bodies become increasingly stronger and ultimately more resilient to declining health and disease.

Only certain plant foods have these nutrients in sufficient quantities to class them as Sirtfoods. As well as matcha, other examples of top Sirtfoods include kale, rocket (arugula), parsley, red onions, strawberries, walnuts, turmeric and cocoa. Because the nutrients in these foods work synergistically, they make great additions in the diet alongside regular consumption of matcha. See also the recipe section from page 52 for a wealth of matcha-rich recipes.

Why is matcha so special?

POW

Glen and Aidan like to refer to matcha as 'green tea on steroids'! Here they outline how matcha smashes standard green tea in terms of its catechin content, and especially its level of EGCG.

One of the frequent findings in green tea research is that to fully realize the benefits of EGCG and the catechins, we need to be drinking multiple cups of green tea a day. Add to that the fact that absorption of EGCG can be hindered when consumed with certain foods, means that to get maximum benefit we might need to drink amounts of green tea that are just not practical for many people.

This leads us on to the beauty of matcha, which is its potency – you don't need to drink lots to gain the health benefits. And as matcha is also a fantastic ingredient for cooking, it's the answer for anyone who wants to reap all the benefits of green tea in the easiest and most convenient way. See the recipe section from page 52 for ideas of how to include matcha in your daily diet.

But wait, there's an added bonus, too. Tea is one of only a few plants that contains L-theanine, and matcha green tea has the advantage of being grown in the shade which means it produces even more L-theanine than standard green tea. L-theanine promotes a mentally relaxed state, reduces nervous system stress and helps stop the mind from racing (see also page 36).

The combination of catechins, low-dose caffeine and L-theanine makes matcha green tea the perfect source of focused energy.

MAXING UP YOUR MATCHA

When it comes to green tea, there can be little doubt that matcha reigns supreme. But to get the maximum bang for your buck, and help you on your way, we've put together our top matcha tips:

OPTIMIZING YOUR MATCHA INTAKE

1. *Ideally opt for organic matcha, which typically contains higher amounts of healthful catechins.*
2. *When making tea, use hot not boiling water (see page 55) to maintain the integrity of the matcha catechins. Off the boil, around 80°C/176°F is perfect.*
3. *Add a squeeze of lemon juice – thanks to its natural acidity it helps to increase the absorption of beneficial green tea compounds.*
4. *Try to drink your matcha tea at least an hour before or two hours after eating food as that will mean you absorb higher amounts of EGCG.*

4 Matcha today

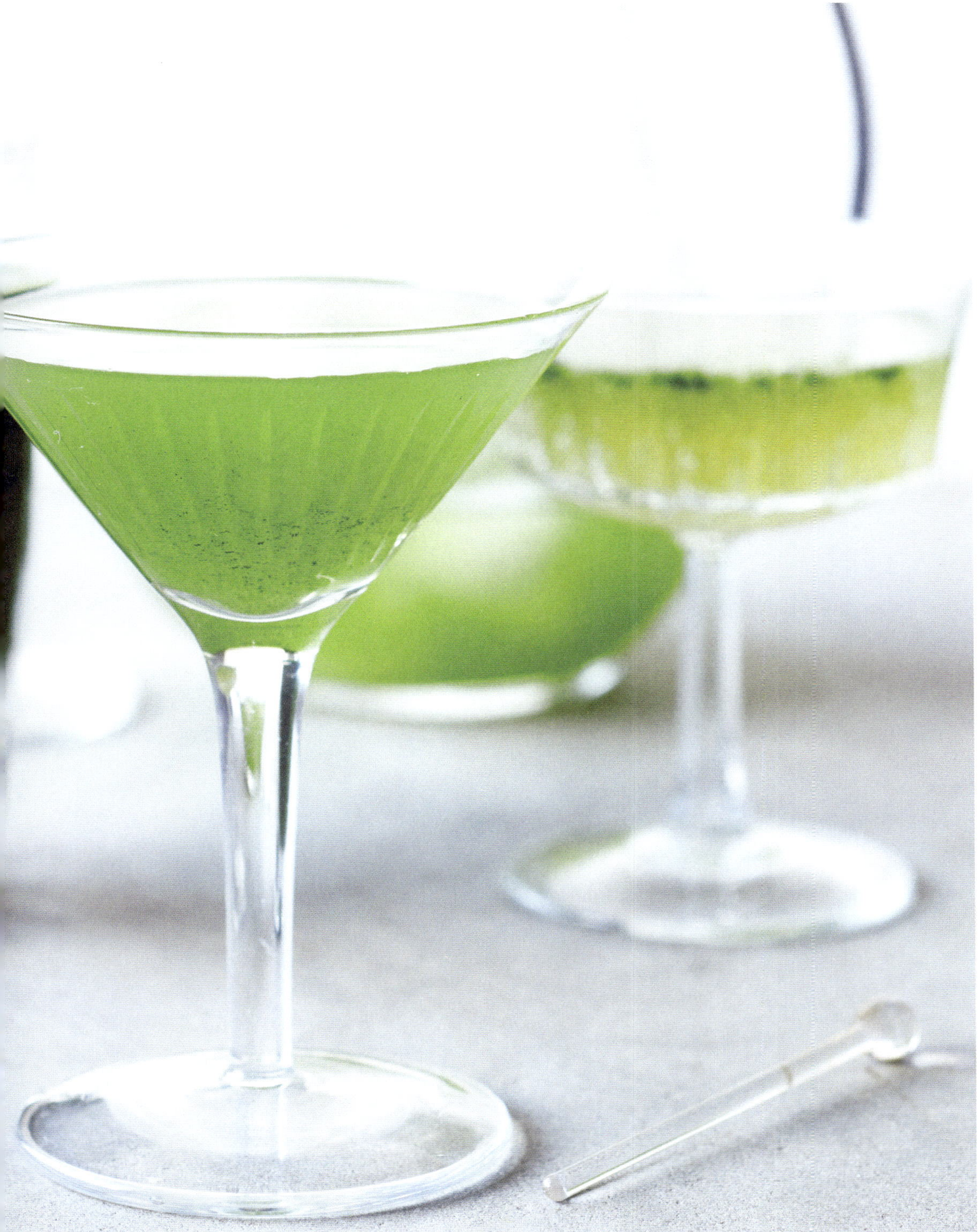

Matcha in the 21st century

Matcha is well and truly part of the culinary experience and social life of Japan. The Japanese incorporate matcha as an ingredient into an amazingly diverse range of drinks and foods, as not only does it have numerous health advantages (see The health benefits, page 32), but its unique flavour can make even the most bland food interesting.

Indeed, as soon as matcha and its umami taste (see opposite) became celebrated in Japan it became an important ingredient in Japanese cuisine. With a distinctive taste, matcha is a high-end flavour to add to anything and everything.

While we understand the long religious significance behind matcha (see The history of matcha, page 8), and ceremonial-grade matcha is traditionally used for the Japanese tea ceremony (see page 12), most of the matcha consumed today is enjoyed for its taste and health benefits. While Buddhist monks have drunk matcha for centuries because of the sustained energy it gives them to aid meditation; today Japanese students consume matcha before exams to give them a boost (and improved results, apparently!).

The rest of the world is now embracing the wonderful, all-natural bright-green brilliance of matcha. There is nothing more satisfying than opening a tin of matcha in front of someone who has never experienced matcha before – the puff of green powder always gets a 'wow!'. This wow factor is why the bright-green powdered tea is now enjoyed the world over. We have all embraced it far beyond the blend of matcha and hot water – adding it to everything from lattes and cocktails to salads and stir-fries.

Nowadays matcha travels all around the world – see page 49 for the best bars, cafés and restaurants to enjoy matcha in. Matcha is also used (and some may think abused!) in all kinds of recipes. See the recipe section from page 52 for how to include matcha in your daily diet.

DRINKING MATCHA AT HOME

First things first – respect the tradition of matcha. While you may not have all the gear (see page 16), whisking matcha into hot water should be experienced and can easily be done at home.

HOW TO DRINK MATCHA: ANY TIME, ANYWHERE

Matcha is incredibly versatile. You can drink it as a hot tea, but you can also add it to fruit juices, smoothies, milk or even a cocktail. See Drinks from page 58 for a wide range of great ideas. It's so easy to get your matcha hit!

1. *Take ½ teaspoon of matcha.*
2. *Add it to your chosen liquid – hot or cold water or milk, fruit juice or smoothie, etc.*
3. *Give it a whisk (electric hand-held whisks work a treat) and enjoy.*

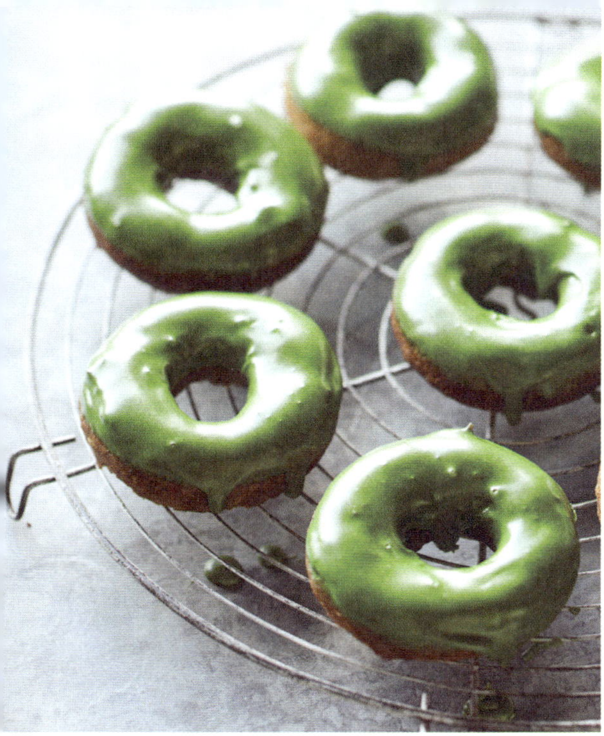

WHAT IS UMAMI?

We all know about the four basic distinct tastes: sweet, sour, bitter and salty, but umami is the fifth main taste. The Japanese chemist Kikunae Ikeda combined 'umai', meaning 'delicious', with 'mi', the word for 'taste', to form 'umami'. Umami has a delicious, savoury, moreish flavour, and can be found in foods such as Parmesan cheese, tomatoes and soy sauce as well as in matcha.

JUST REMEMBER...

As an ingredient, matcha works particularly well with creamy, indulgent flavours. If you are enjoying matcha just for its health benefits we hopefully don't need to spell it out that the matcha goodness may be compromised if you enjoy it in an indulgent, cream-topped form!

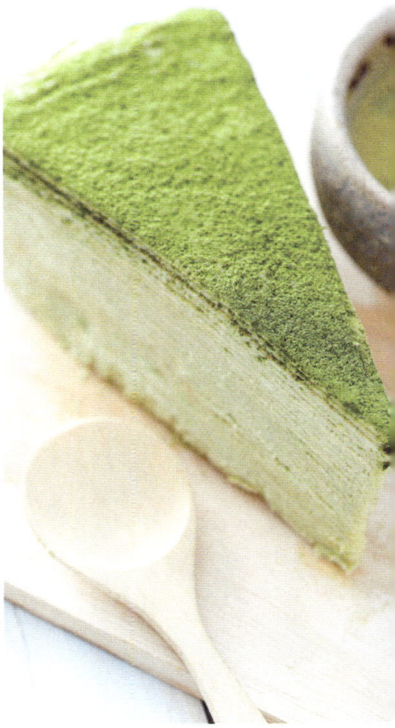

MATCHA AS A FOOD

Matcha as a drink is only the beginning – because it is a powder you can add it to your porridge, yoghurt, cakes, desserts, soups . . . any number of different foods. We have given you lots of ideas for creating your own matcha meals (see page 52 onwards).

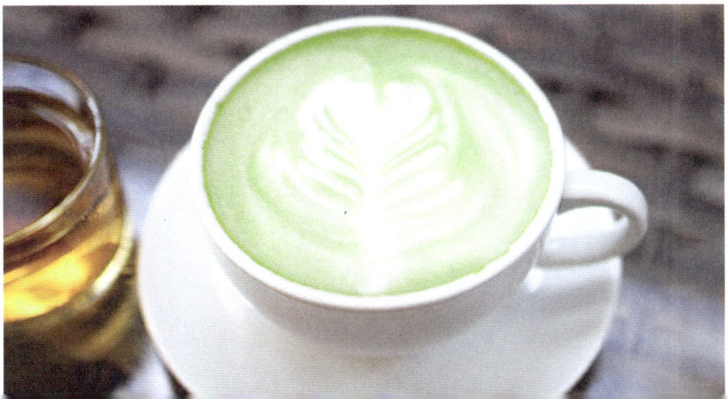

MATCHA FOR ANY MEAL

Matcha is everywhere – and in everything – in Japan. But beyond Japan, the taste for matcha has really grown over the last 10 or so years and matcha can now be enjoyed around the world. The US sales alone of matcha increased more than 50 per cent in 2014 as the 'matcha wave' really began to take off.

Below are some of the top ways to try matcha in drinks and foods.

MATCHA ICE CREAM

This is delicious if made well, with top-quality matcha and ice cream. We love the creaminess and vivid green colour of Coconut and matcha ice cream (see page 163); or why not try the Matcha mochi ice cream balls (see page 167) for a taste of Japan at home.
Worth a visit: Japan Ice OUCA, 1 Chome-6-6 Ebisu, Tokyo, 150-0013, Japan. (www.ice-ouca.com)
Tombo Japanese Café and Matcha Bar, 29 Thurloe Place, London SW7 2HQ, England. (www.tombocafe.com)

MATCHA CAKES AND DESSERTS

Sweet little treats can be found all over Japan, where bright-green matcha jellies and indulgent cakes are common. Why not try our Mini matcha cheesecakes on page 154 or the Matcha breakfast muffins on page 84.

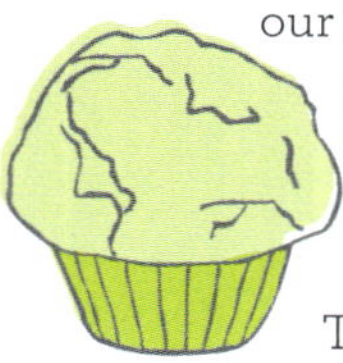

Worth a visit: Chachanoma, 5-13-14 Jingumae, Shibuya-ku, Tokyo, 150-0001, Japan. (www.chachanoma.com)
Nana's Green Tea, LaQua Building 3F, 1-1-1 Kasuga, Bunkyo-ku, Tokyo, Japan. (www.nanasgreentea.com)

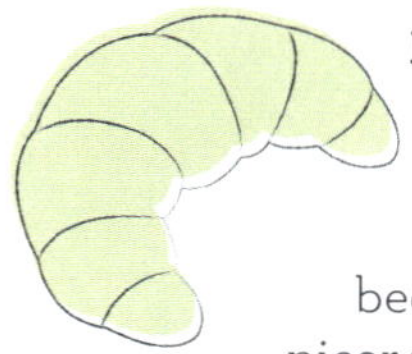

MATCHA PASTRIES

As the Western diet and the Japanese diet merge, green matcha pastries have been created. What could be nicer than a Matcha croissant (see page 86) or indulgent Matcha ring doughnuts (see page 142)?
Worth a visit: Sadaharu Aoki is a Japanese pastry chef who lives in Paris, France, and has created numerous matcha-based treats. He has a number of outlets across Japan and in Paris, France. (www.sadaharuaoki.jp/en/)
Aki Boulangerie, a specialist French-Japanese bakery, is at 16 rue Sainte-Anne, 75001, Paris, France. (www.akiparis.fr)

MATCHA LATTE

The matcha latte is a global favourite (see recipes on page 62), and can generally be found on the menu of any café or restaurant serving matcha.
Worth a visit: Starbucks have a number of matcha-themed drinks – both juices and hot drinks – on their menu. These are a long way from the bamboo whisk and porcelain bowl but are worth trying (www.starbucks.com).
Bibble and Sip, 253 W 51st St, New York, NY 10019, USA. (www.bibbleandsip.com)

MATCHA BEER

Green beer, including a number of matcha-based beers, plus interesting food can be enjoyed in the matcha beer garden in the tea-centred restaurant, 1899.

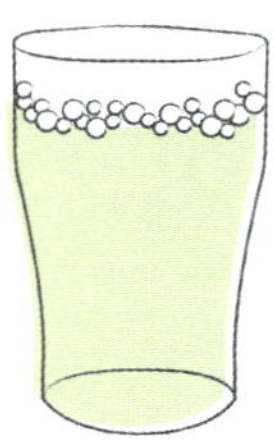

Worth a visit: 1899, 3–4 Kanda-surugadai Chiyoda-ku, Tokyo, 101-0062, Japan. (www.1899.jp/ochanomizu/en/)

WEIRD . . . OR WONDERFULLY GREEN?

Matcha popcorn, Oreos, KitKats, ice lollies or truffles anyone? Here are some interesting matcha-infused treats.

Matcha crisps

Salt and vinegar, cheese and onion or matcha crisps? Which do you fancy? The largest Japanese snack food maker, Koike-ya, have sourced a fine matcha from Uji and infused it into their potato crisps to make a high-end Japanese snack.

Matcha on toast

Although some people may find the distinctive green colour of matcha bread slightly unnerving, you can even top it with a matcha milk spread (or 'milk jam') – the green equivalent to a chocolate spread. Lots of food companies produce the spread, or you can easily make it at home. A bright-green spread to go on your bright-green toast. Delicious.

Matcha booze

We all love a cocktail blended with matcha (see our Green martini and Mint fizz cocktails on page 70). In Japan you can buy matcha sake, the ultimate Japanese drink. The matcha is infused at the point of production so the sake has a very strong matcha flavour. New to the market is kahluha and matcha, one to try (perhaps!).

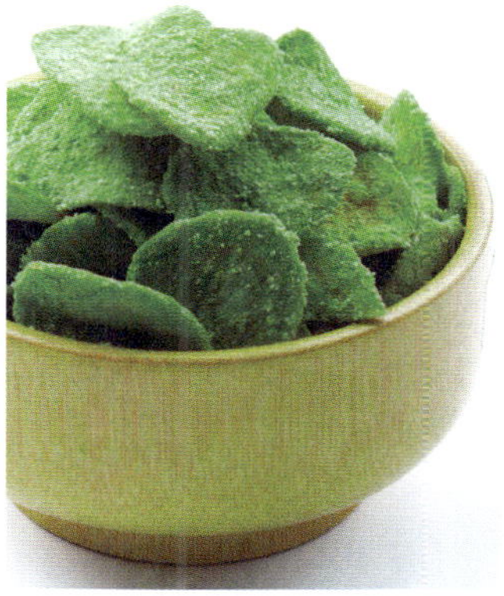

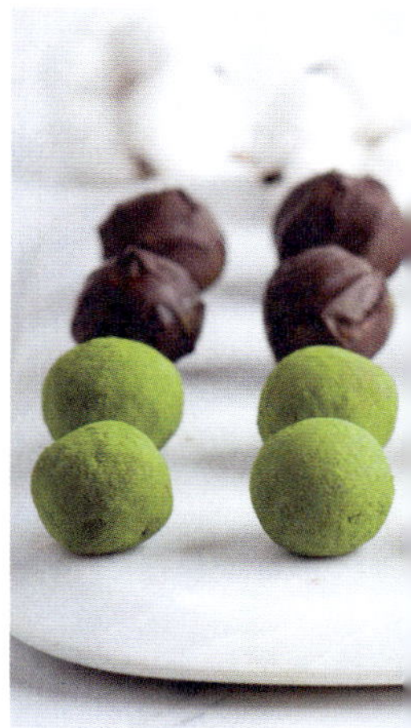

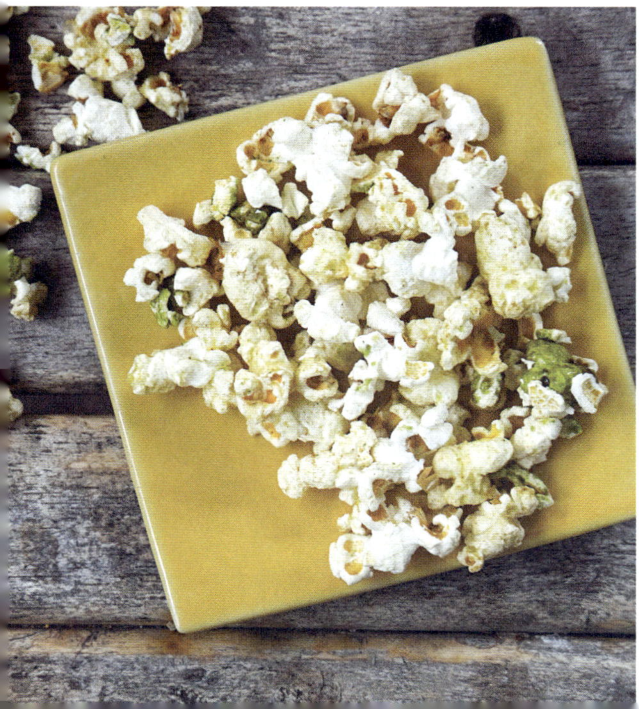

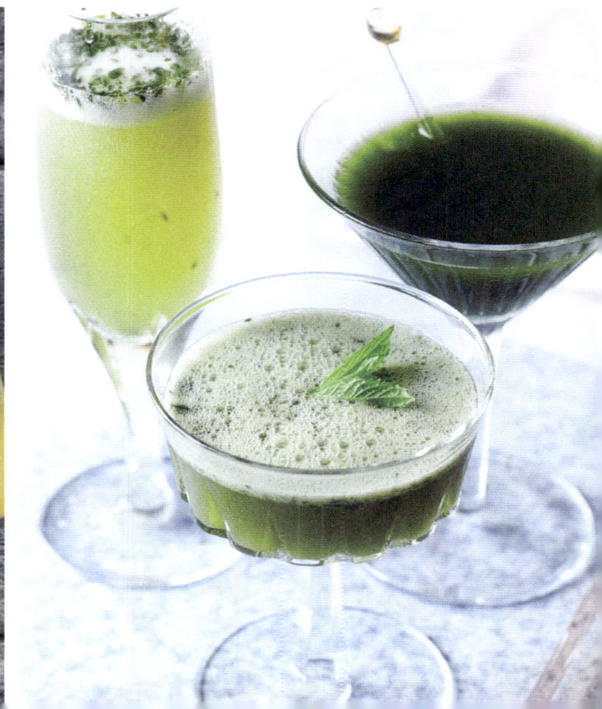

WHERE TO EXPERIENCE THE TEA CEREMONY

For many people, experiencing the tea ceremony while on a visit to Japan is a highlight of their trip. Most of the tea houses given here are in Kyoto, which is the traditional home of the tea ceremony, but with careful research you will be able to find tea houses all over Japan where you will be able to experience an authentic tea ceremony.

Camellia, Kyoto

With two locations in Kyoto, Camellia's super-calm Flower tea house is located on Ninenzaka steps between Gion and Kiyomizu Temple, in one of Kyoto's historical preservation neighbourhoods. A great place to experience a mesmerizing ceremony. Camellia's Garden tea house is in the west of Kyoto, situated amongst peaceful gardens and moments away from Ryoan-ji – the world-renowned Zen temple and rock garden.

Flower tea house, 349 Masuya-cho, Higashiyama-ku, Kyoto.
Garden tea house 18 Ryoanji Ikenoshita-cho, Ukyo-ku, Kyoto.
(www.tea-kyoto.com)

Grand Tea Room Ju-An, Kyoto

Just 10 minutes from Kyoto Station, this authentic tea house is the real deal. Located in an architectural gem in historic Kyoto, this elegant tea house is set in a typical Japanese garden. Here you can learn all about the rituals of the ceremony, and practise the Japanese tea ceremony with an English-speaking host.

508 Shiokojicho, Shimogyo Ward, Kyoto.
(www.teaceremonykyoto.com)

Yuuhisai Koudoukan, Kyoto

This is a premium tea house experience. Held in an historic building surrounded by a tranquil garden. The utensils used are all ceremonial grade and often highly prized works of art. They look to the seasons for their chosen tools as well as edible offerings.

524–1 Mototsuchimikado-cho, Kamichoja-machi dori, Shinmachi Higashi-iru, Kamigyo-ku, Kyoto.
(www.kodo-kan.com/english/tea)

Ran Hotei, Kyoto

Set in a 100-year-old Kyoto townhouse, this elegant tea house is just 10 minutes south of Nijo Castle. Experience the ceremony with Canadian tea master Randy Channell Soei at this exquisite tea house and gallery.

64 Kamikawara, Sanjo Omiya, Kyoto.
(www.ranhotei.com)

Taiho-an, Uji

It is worth the trip south of Kyoto to experience a tea ceremony in the tea-growing region of Uji. A serene setting to learn about the culture surrounding tea production and the ceremony.

1–5 Uji-togawa, Uji, Kyoto.
(www.kyoto-uji-kankou.or.jp/taihoan-en)

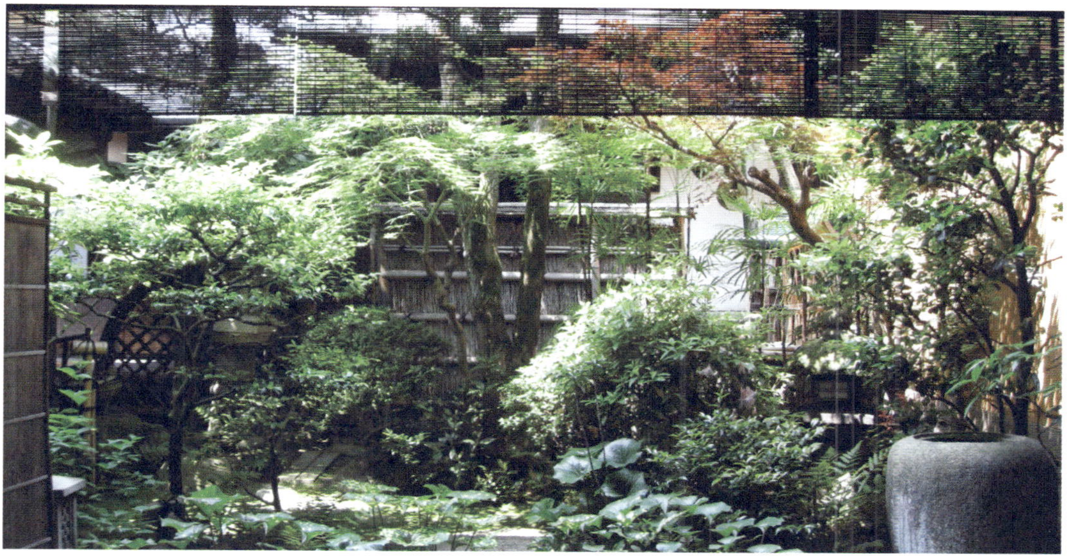

Hotel Chinzanso, Tokyo

Set amidst the bustle of Tokyo, this 'urban oasis' has tranquil and historic tea rooms set in the middle of a stunning garden, which is in full bloom all year round. The tea ceremony led by the hotel's resident tea master is not to be missed.
10-8, Sekiguchi 2-chome, Bunkyo-ku, Tokyo.
(www.hotel-chinzanso-tokyo.com)

d:matcha, Kyoto

Not a traditional tea ceremony, but the thought and effort that is put in at this modern tea farm makes it well worth a visit. They offer a hands-on experience of many aspects of the farming and production process as well as tasting flights of their teas (a range of green teas, including matcha).
Gonose-142 Yubune, Wazuka, Kyoto.
(www.dmatcha.com)

Tondaya, Kyoto

This atmospheric tea house is located in an ancient merchant house or Machiya. Tondaya was registered as National Cultural Heritage site in 1999 and is a lifestyle museum. As well as experiencing the tea ceremony you can hire kimonos, take a tour of the historic building and learn all about traditional Japanese arts such as calligraphy and origami.
697 Ishiyakushicho, Kamigyo-ku Kyoto.
(www.tondaya.co.jp/english)

THE BEST OF MATCHA WORLDWIDE

Matcha has been a feature on menus in hipster cafés and Japanese restaurants outside Japan for some time. It is now present on the menu of some mainstream chains, and a number of dedicated matcha bars are opening up outside Japan. These are great places to experiment with matcha creations. See below for where to experience the best of matcha around the world.

In Australia

Oh!Matcha is an authentic, Japanese-style café in the Sydney central business district, providing a delicious selection of matcha drinks – from floats to frappés – as well as a traditional-modern Japanese menu.
Shop 11, 501 George Street, Sydney 2000 NSW.
(www.ohmatcha.com.au)

Little Rogue is a coffee house featuring matcha lattes and amazing latte art.
12 Drewery Lane, Melbourne, Victoria 3000.
(www.littlerogue.com.au)

Matcha-ya is a cafe and bar on the edge of Sydney's Chinatown offering a wide range of beverages and sweet treats (a matcha jiggly cat pudding is particularly adorable) alongside delicious savouries. They take their matcha seriously though, sourcing it direct from Japan by attending tea auctions four times a year.
05/10 Steam Mill Lane, Sydney 2000 NSW.
(www.matchaya.com.au)

In Canada

Uncle Tetsu's Japanese Cheesecake Café is a vibrant café featuring a wide range of smoothies, bright-green desserts and sweet treats on its menu. Famous for the Uncle Tetsu Matcha Cheesecake.
Several locations across Canada. Find your nearest online.
(www.uncletetsu-ca.com)

Matcha Matcha has a few locations across in Toronto and as the name might suggest, there is a total dedication to matcha. Despite one or two deviations for those that absolutely cannot go without their coffee fix, this café has a focused menu and is definitely one for the matcha lovers.
407 Church St, Toronto, ON M5B 1J2.
(www.matchamatcha.ca)

In Germany

This German version of the American café chain **House of Small Wonder** opened in Berlin in December 2014. With numerous Japanese influences, the menu features matcha heavily, while the matcha cappucino is something else!
Auguststraße 11–13, 10117 Berlin.
(www.houseofsmallwonder.de)

In Hong Kong

Winstons Coffee (*pictured opposite*) is a popular addition to the matcha coffee scene (and in the evening – the cocktail scene). Try a matcha latte with a matcha bagel – delicious! With four locations across Hong Kong to choose from, you can easily find your matcha fix.
Shop 4, G/F Rich Court, 213 Queens Road West, Sai Ying Pun.
(www.winstonscoffee.com)

In Singapore

With over 160 years of history, and seven shops across Singapore, **Tsujiri** serves the most amazing matcha ice cream desserts, along with a wide range of hot matcha beverages.
6 Eu Tong Sen Street #01-74 The Central Singapore 059817.
(www.tsujiri.sg)

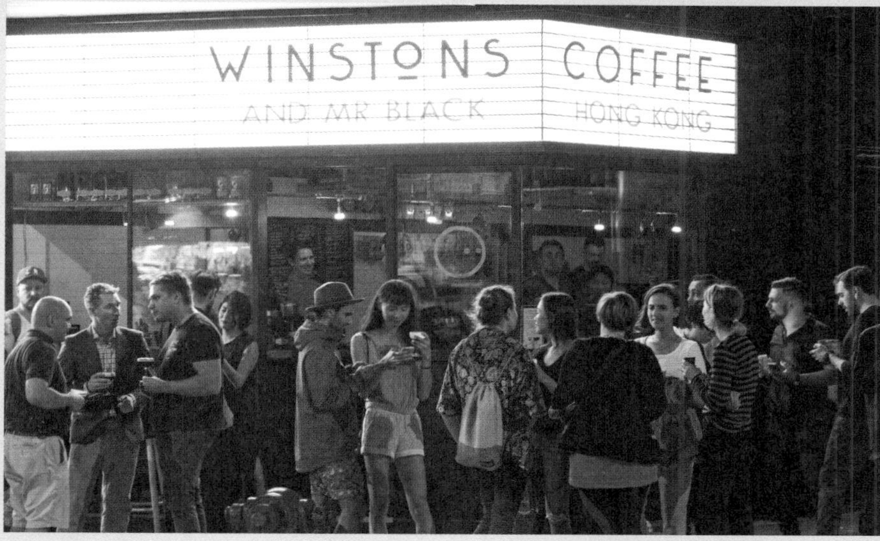

In the UK

TSUJIRI has been producing matcha in Japan since 1860. Now serving it globally, every cup of matcha from TSUJIRI comes with a rich history. Thankfully there are several locations across the UK. Find your nearest online.
(www.tsujiri.co.uk)

Moksha Caffe were very early adopters of the matcha trend and are an excellent spot for brunch.
4–5 York Place, Brighton, BN1 4GU.
(www.mokshacaffe.co.uk)

JENKI have had an amazing start since opening their doors in 2021, with sites popping up in some of London's hottest spots. Their focus is on the matcha craft alongside good-looking, wholesome beverages.
43 Brushfield Street, E1 6AA.
(www.jenki.co.uk)

Godshot Studio in Glasgow isn't your typical coffee shop. A lifestyle and design store that creates the most stunning coffee, tea and patisserie. The matcha menu is a delight but the store is well worth a visit beyond sampling some of their green offerings.
1143 Pollokshaws Road, Shawlands, Glasgow G41 3YH.
(www.mygodshot.com)

In the USA

Matchaful weaves together ancient wisdom and healthful ingredients to create a menu that has a wide selection of matcha offerings. With a focus on nutrition as well as traditions, you'll leave feeling fab after a visit to one of their locations.
184 Prince Street, New York, NY 10012.
(www.matchaful.com)

When **12matcha** opened, it was a big deal. They have a cutting-edge take when it comes to making matcha. Working with scientists and artisans to hone their craft, they even installed specialist water tanks with custom filtration to brew the tea.
54 Bond Street, New York, NY 10012.
(www.12matcha.com)

Tea Master Matcha Café and Green Tea Shop is less concerned with the futuristic aspects of tea making and has managed to keep things simple. With a pared-down menu and no gimmicks, everything is whisked with a dedication to the craft of matcha. Here, the focus is the tea.
450E 2nd Street, Los Angeles, CA 90012.
(www.teamastermatcha.com)

Matcha recipes

Choosing, storing and preparing matcha 54

The matcha challenge 56

Drinks 58

Breakfast 72

Snacks 92

Main meals 108

Bakes 132

Desserts 150

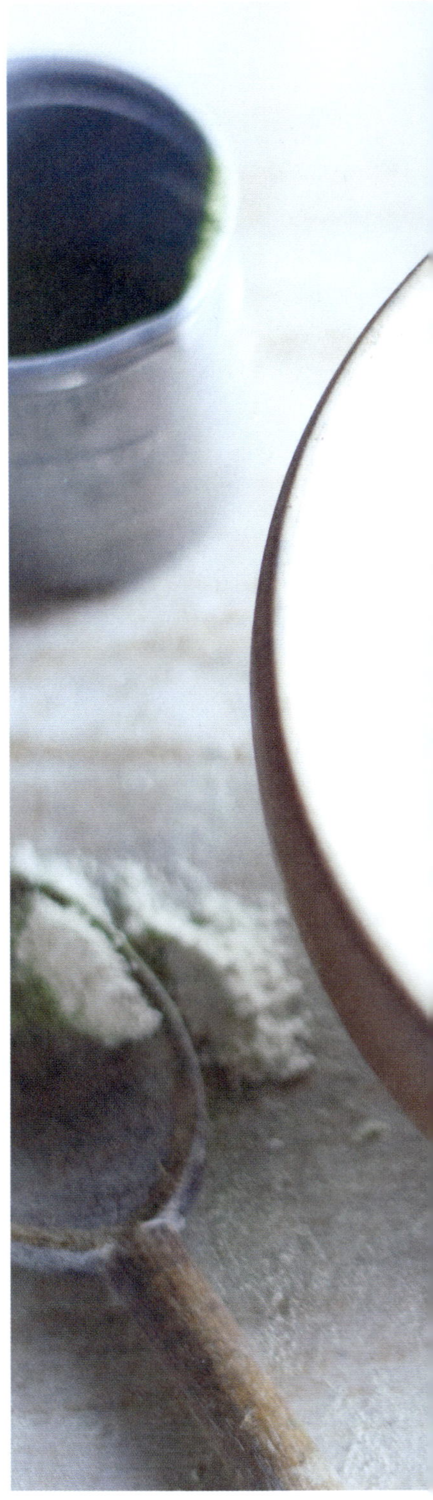

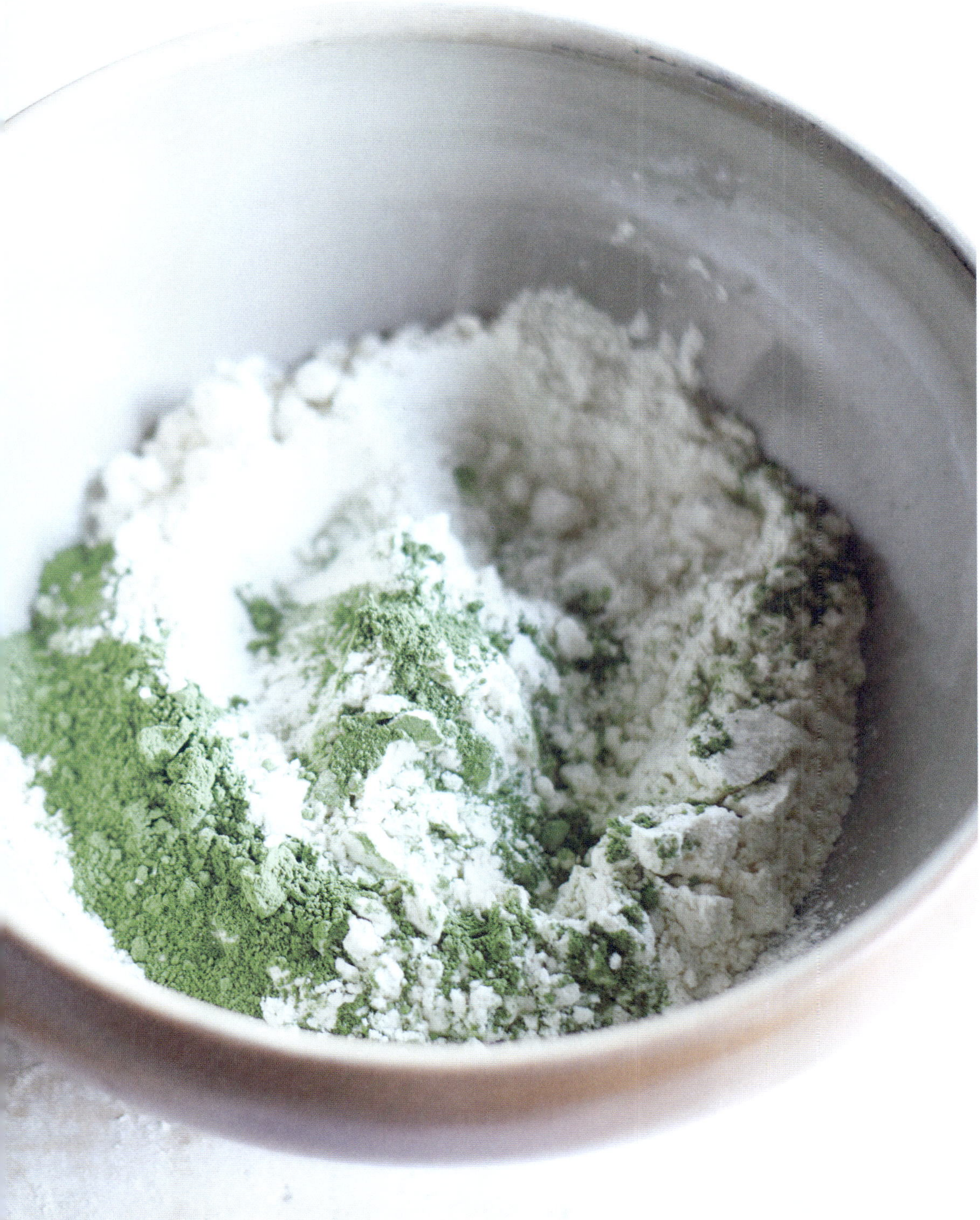

Choosing, storing and preparing matcha

Matcha is a wonderful ingredient, but not all matcha is the same. Like most foods and drinks, there is a wide range available. See below for what to look for in top-quality matcha, and how to look after it once you have purchased it.

Look

You want a bright-green, rich, fresh-looking powder. This indicates that the stems and veins have been removed, and only the quality 'fleshy' parts of the leaves have been used.

Smell

Giving the matcha a good sniff tells you the quality of the matcha – a sweet, vegetable, fresh smell means good stuff!

On the go?
Add a matcha sachet to your drink bottle, shake and drink!

Taste

A good-quality matcha tastes good... it's as simple as that. It should have a thick, sweet, umami taste (see page 45), with no astringency or bitterness. While the taste of matcha itself is unusual, it should never be unpleasant.

Touch

If you compare a quality matcha with a low-grade green tea powder you can feel the difference. Pour out a small pile of each powder onto some paper. Press your finger into each and drag it outwards (almost like you are painting a finger picture). The good-quality matcha feels like face cream – thick and smooth. The green tea powder will feel more grainy and dry.

Appearance

The matcha should be a rich, bright, deep green colour when brewed.

Storage

Now that you have invested in the finest matcha, make sure you look after it. Matcha is processed in a cool, dark room to keep it super fresh, so keeping it in a cool, dark place, such as the fridge, is ideal.

Light isn't great for matcha, so put the lid on quickly after you have taken the matcha out. If the matcha is not going to be consumed for a while, then store it in the freezer.

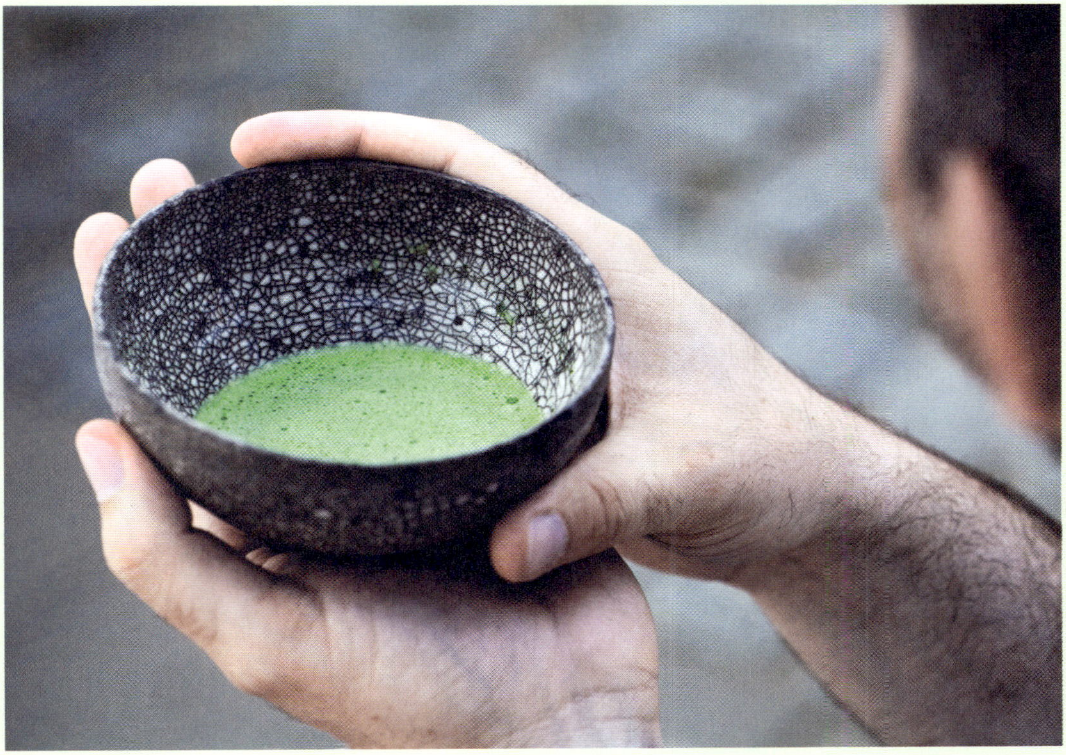

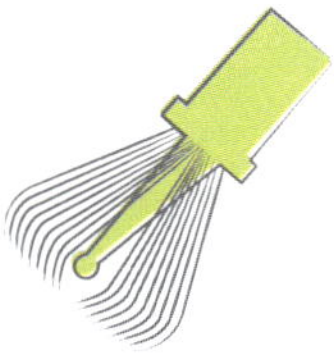

HOW TO MAKE MATCHA THE TRADITIONAL WAY

The classic way to make matcha tea is to whisk it into hot water using a bamboo whisk, then serve it in a bowl, as the Japanese do.

Alternatively, although not quite as authentic, you can use an electric hand-held whisk or milk frother if you don't have a bamboo whisk.

1. Add a scoop (about ½ teaspoon), of matcha to your bowl.
2. Add a small amount of warm (but not boiling) water – if the water is too hot it will burn the leaves.
3. Whisk the matcha and water together using a bamboo whisk.
4. Top up with warm water and enjoy straight away.

The matcha challenge

We've heard all about matcha's superpowers, and lots of people tell us how drinking matcha has made them feel more energized and focused.

When teapigs first brought matcha to the UK, people were invited to take the matcha challenge: to drink matcha every day for two weeks and see how sprightly they felt. The results were amazing. We first launched the challenge in 2016 and had 700 people take part. An amazing 81 per cent of participants said they felt more energized.

If you'd like to give it a go, we've put together this calendar to help you enjoy your matcha in many different ways; or check out the recipes that follow.

THE MATCHA CHALLENGE CALENDAR

DAY 1

Welcome to the first day of the matcha challenge.

Enjoy a Glorious green or Beautiful berry juice (see page 60) for a real health kick.

DAY 2

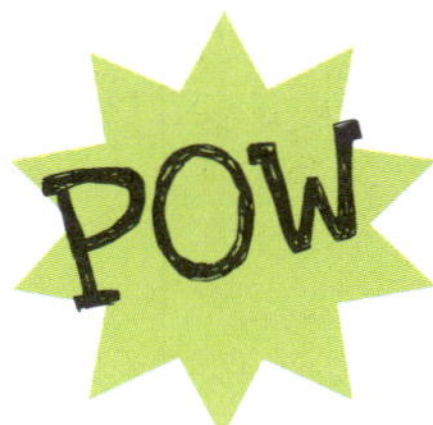

Start the day properly with Matcha eggs Florentine (see page 90) or Matcha granola with berries (see page 82). Yum.

DAY 3

Unlike coffee, you won't get a rush of energy and then a crash with matcha. It's all about slow release . . .

Relax and enjoy a cup of matcha tea mid-morning.

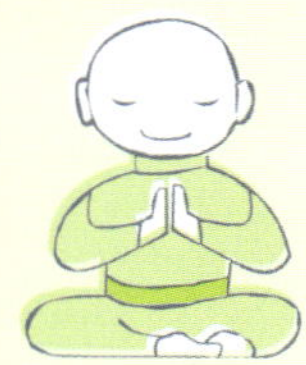

DAY 4

99%

of people would recommend matcha to a friend.

Raw matcha coconut fudge bites (see page 106) are ideal for sharing with friends.

DAY 5

Enjoy a tea break with a friend.

Knock up an Almond matcha latte or a White chocolate matcha latte (see page 62).

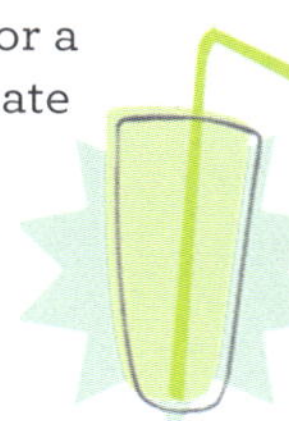

DAY 6

In a rush? Take your matcha on the go.

Simply add matcha to your water bottle, shake and drink!

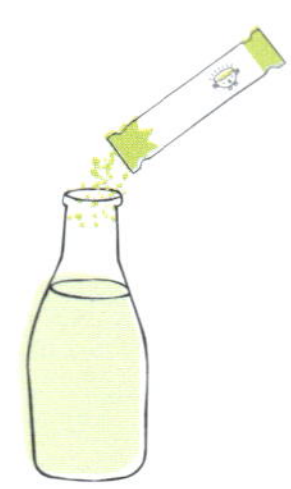

DAY 7

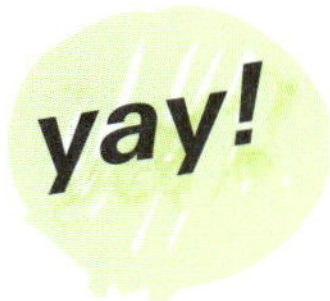

You're halfway through!
Treat time . . .

Matcha blondies (see page 140) are decadent and moreish.

DAY 8

We love that matcha is so versatile you can enjoy it at any meal.

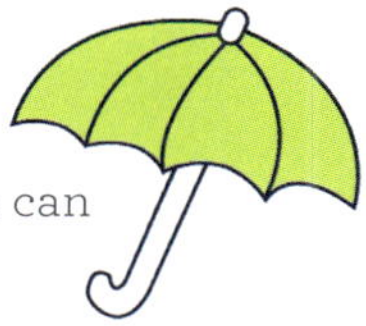

Matcha poached salmon, broccoli and chickpea salad (see page 112) makes a perfect power-packed lunch.

DAY 9

81%

of people felt more energized after having matcha for two weeks.

The Hazelnut and vanilla smoothie (see page 74) is packed with flavour and goodness.

DAY 10

Matcha for dinner? Why not?!

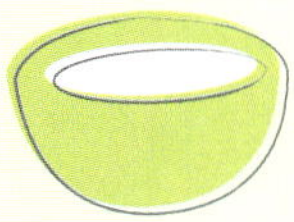

Chicken, turmeric, matcha and pepper casserole (see page 126) is wonderfully spicy.

DAY 11

Matcha tastes great with citrus. Why not try:

A refreshing Matcha lemonade (see page 68).

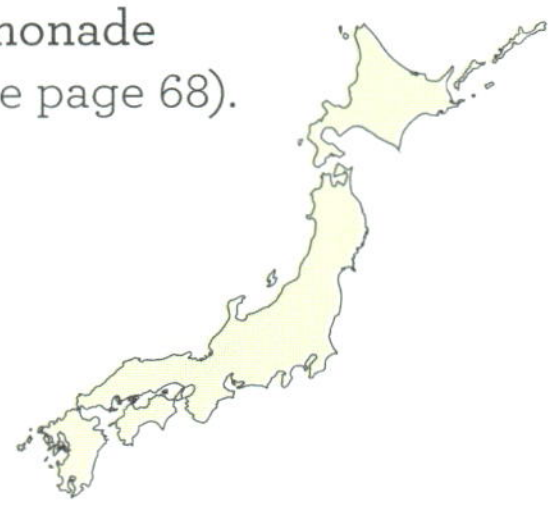

DAY 12

Healthy breakfast!

Try the yummy Matcha overnight oats (see page 79).

DAY 13

One day to go – it's matcha cocktail time!

What do you fancy?

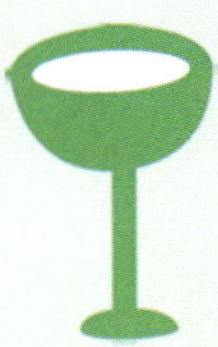

A Green martini or maybe a zingy Mint fizz cocktail (see page 70)?

DAY 14

Yay! You completed the matcha challenge . . .

Coconut and matcha cupcakes (see page 139) . . . it is a celebration after all!

Drinks

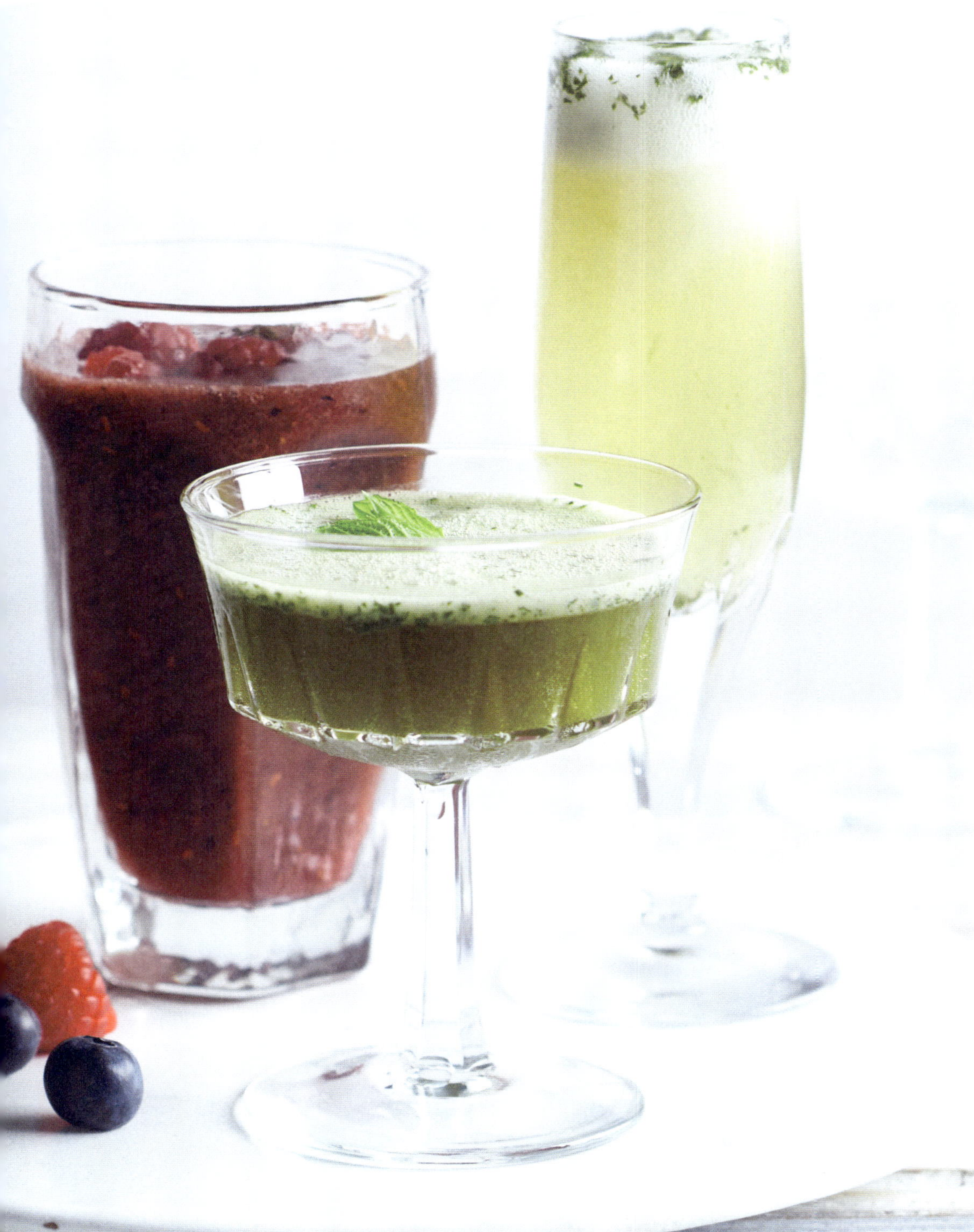

Matcha juices

We teamed up with the highly-regarded nutritionists Aidan Goggins and Glen Matten to create some super-healthy recipes, including two of these delicious juices. Here they tell us why these juices are so great for you. To make these vibrant juices, simply place all the ingredients in a blender and blend until smooth. Serve immediately over ice.

Peach and apple juice

This juice is fresh, sweet and summery, and the addition of Greek yoghurt makes it feel delightfully indulgent.

SERVES 1

1 peach, peeled and stoned (pitted)
100ml (½ cup) apple juice
1 tbsp Greek yoghurt
½ tsp matcha powder
squeeze of runny honey

Glorious green juice

'Go green with the brassica queen! Packed with vitamins C, K and folate as well as polyphenols and immune-boosting beta-carotene, kale is a nutrient powerhouse, which when combined with matcha makes for a health blockbuster. The addition of banana gives it an irresistible creaminess.'

SERVES 1

1 banana
2 handfuls of kale
juice of 1 lime
100ml (½ cup) apple juice
½ tsp matcha powder

Beautiful berry juice

'We love berries and their bumper supply of healthful anthocyanins, the pigments that give berries their colour and have potent benefits in warding off obesity, diabetes and heart disease, as well as boosting bone density and brain health.'

SERVES 1

5 large strawberries
10 raspberries
10 blueberries
100ml (½ cup) apple juice
5 mint leaves
2 sprigs of basil
½ tsp matcha powder

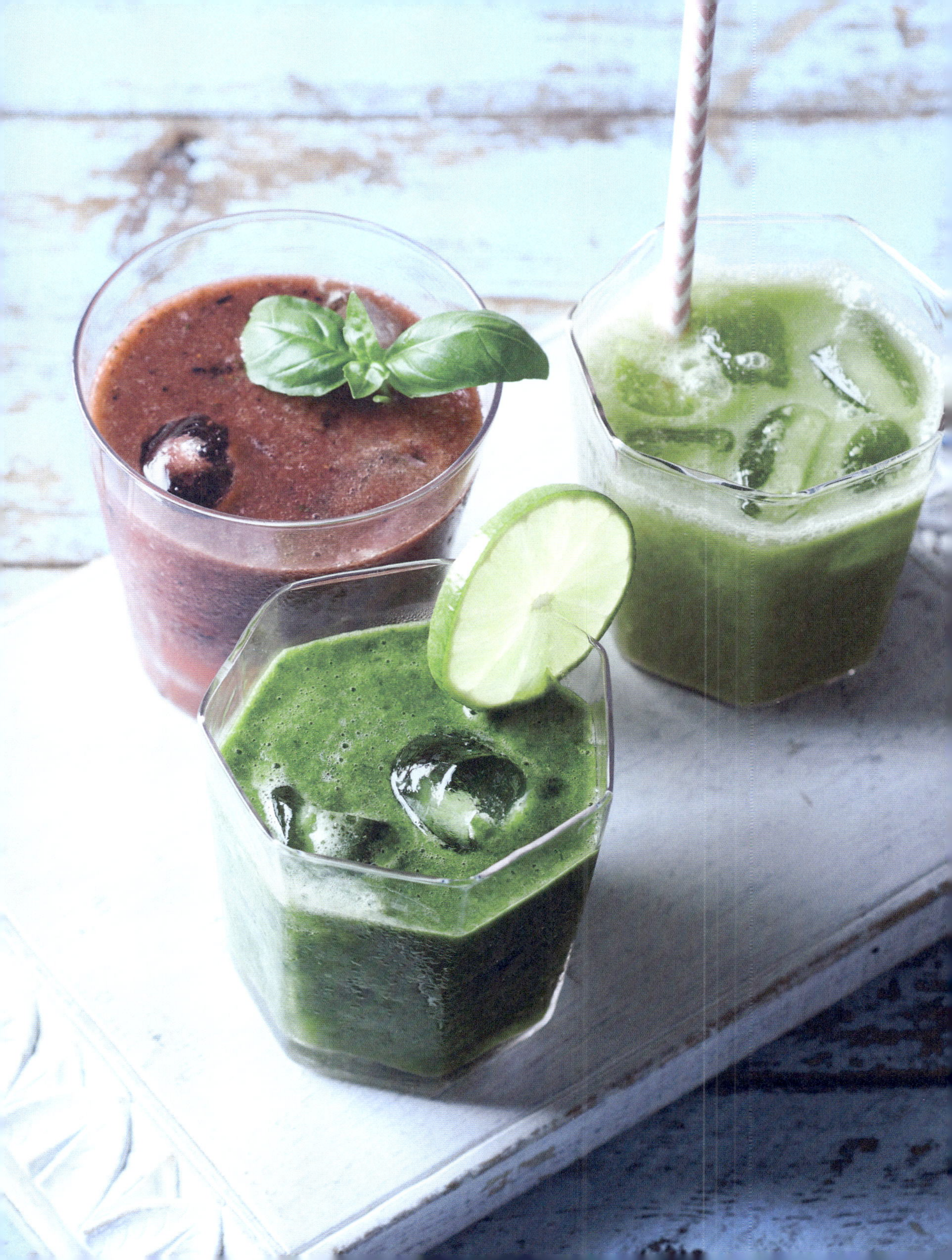

Almond matcha latte

This is equally delicious made with hazelnut or coconut milk. If using cow's milk, choose semi-skimmed (skim) because the matcha flavour comes through better.

SERVES 1

½ tsp matcha powder
a little hot water
squeeze of agave syrup
½ tsp ground cinnamon
½ tsp ground nutmeg
¼ tsp vanilla powder
300ml (1¼ cups) unsweetened almond milk

1 Put the matcha powder in a mug and add a little hot (but not boiling) water. Whisk to make a paste – we use a small hand-held battery-operated whisk.

2 Add the agave syrup, cinnamon, nutmeg and vanilla powder and stir or whisk again.

3 Heat the almond milk and whisk to make frothy. A hand-held whisk works well, or if you have a coffee machine with a steamer, you can use that.

4 Add the milk to the matcha paste and enjoy the yumminess!

White chocolate matcha latte

Matcha tastes simply amazing with white chocolate, and this tasty latte is perfect for an indulgent treat. Just add a slice of Chocolate layer cake (see page 134) or a Matcha macaron (see page 144) and you'll be in matcha heaven.

SERVES 1

100ml (½ cup) whipping (heavy) cream
30g (1oz) white chocolate
200ml (1 cup) semi-skimmed (skim) milk
¼ tsp vanilla powder
½ tsp matcha powder, plus extra for sprinkling

1 Whip the cream and set aside.

2 Melt the white chocolate in a saucepan with the milk and vanilla powder.

3 Add the matcha powder to the saucepan and whisk until smooth, then pour into a mug.

4 Pile the whipped cream on top of the latte.

5 Add a sprinkling of matcha powder for fun and green-ness!

Note
The Almond matcha latte is amazing iced. Just make a paste with a little cold almond milk (instead of hot water), add the agave and spices and top with more almond milk and ice.

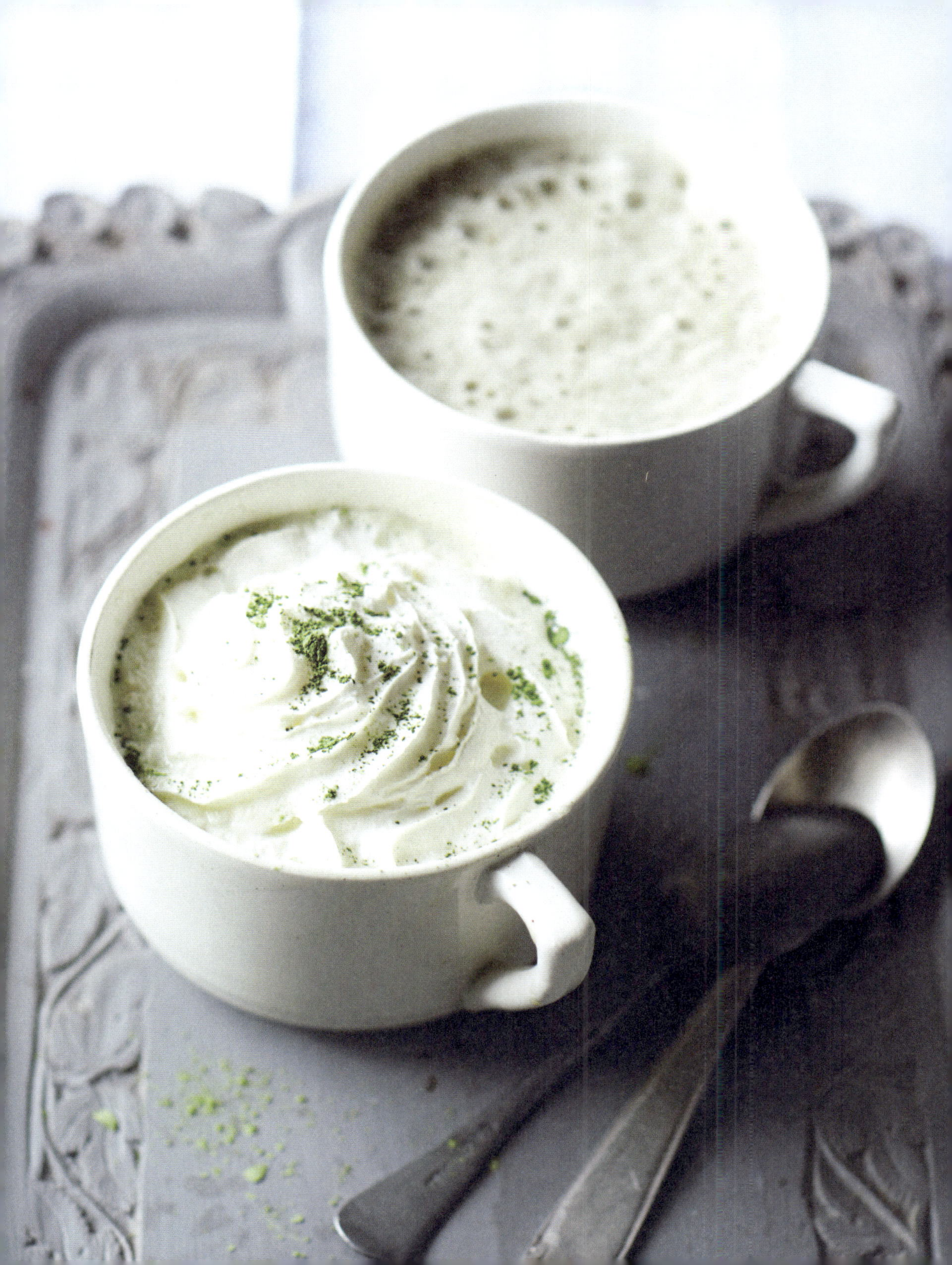

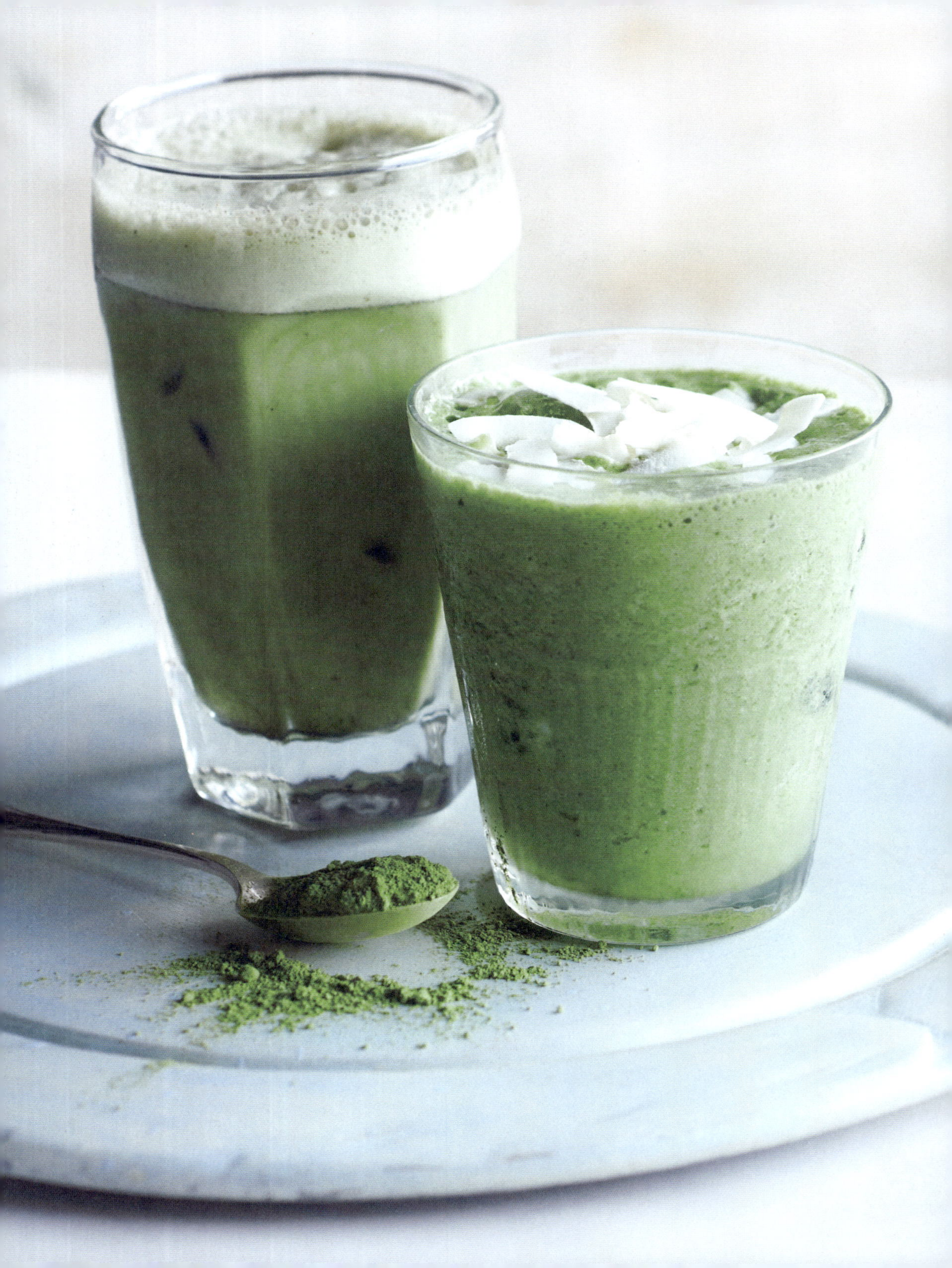

Dairy-free almond and matcha frappé

Almonds and matcha are a great combination in this refreshing frappé. Make sure you use a good-quality almond milk with no added sugar, and you'll get a delicate sweetness from the almonds as well as the burst of matcha goodness.

SERVES 1

200ml (1 cup) almond milk
½ tsp matcha powder
¼ tsp vanilla powder
2 ice cubes, plus extra for serving

1 Add the almond milk, matcha powder, vanilla powder and 2 ice cubes to a blender.

2 Blend until smooth, then pour over ice and serve immediately.

Matcha coconut teashake

You can make this super-simple teashake with any ice cream you fancy, but our favourite flavours are coconut, vanilla or ginger. The coconut flakes on top make this even yummier, or for the ultimate drink use white chocolate sprinkles.

SERVES 1

100ml (½ cup) skimmed (skim) milk
2–3 scoops of coconut ice cream
1 tsp matcha powder
coconut milk, to thin the consistency, if desired
coconut flakes (optional)

1 Put the milk and ice cream into a blender and blend.

2 Add the matcha powder and blend again.

3 Depending on how thick you like it, add coconut milk and blend again until you reach the desired thickness.

4 Pour into a glass, sprinkle with coconut flakes if you wish, drink and grin!

White chocolate and matcha milkshake

Yum, yum, yum! Creamy vanilla and white chocolate mixed with matcha is an indulgent and dreamy combination. Dress it up or down as you wish, varying the decoration depending on your mood.

SERVES 1

100ml (½ cup) whipping (heavy) cream
25g (1oz) white chocolate chips, plus extra to serve
½ tsp vanilla sugar
300ml (1¼ cups) semi-skimmed (skim) milk
½ tsp matcha powder
squeeze of runny honey

1 Whip the cream and set aside.

2 Melt the chocolate chips in a saucepan over a low heat.

3 Mix the vanilla sugar into the milk.

4 Add the milk, matcha powder and honey to the melted chocolate mixture and blend or whisk.

5 Pour into a glass. Garnish with the whipped cream and reserved chocolate chips, and serve immediately.

Vanilla matcha milkshake

Guilt-free, this dairy-free milkshake tastes lovely and creamy and is packed with goodness from the matcha, banana and almond milk. For variety, experiment with other kinds of milk – coconut milk works particularly well.

SERVES 1

1 banana, frozen
115ml (½ cup) unsweetened almond milk
½ tsp matcha powder
½ tsp vanilla powder, plus extra to serve
3 handfuls of ice cubes
squeeze of runny honey

1 Add all the ingredients to a blender and blend until smooth.

2 Serve with a sprinkling of vanilla powder and some ice.

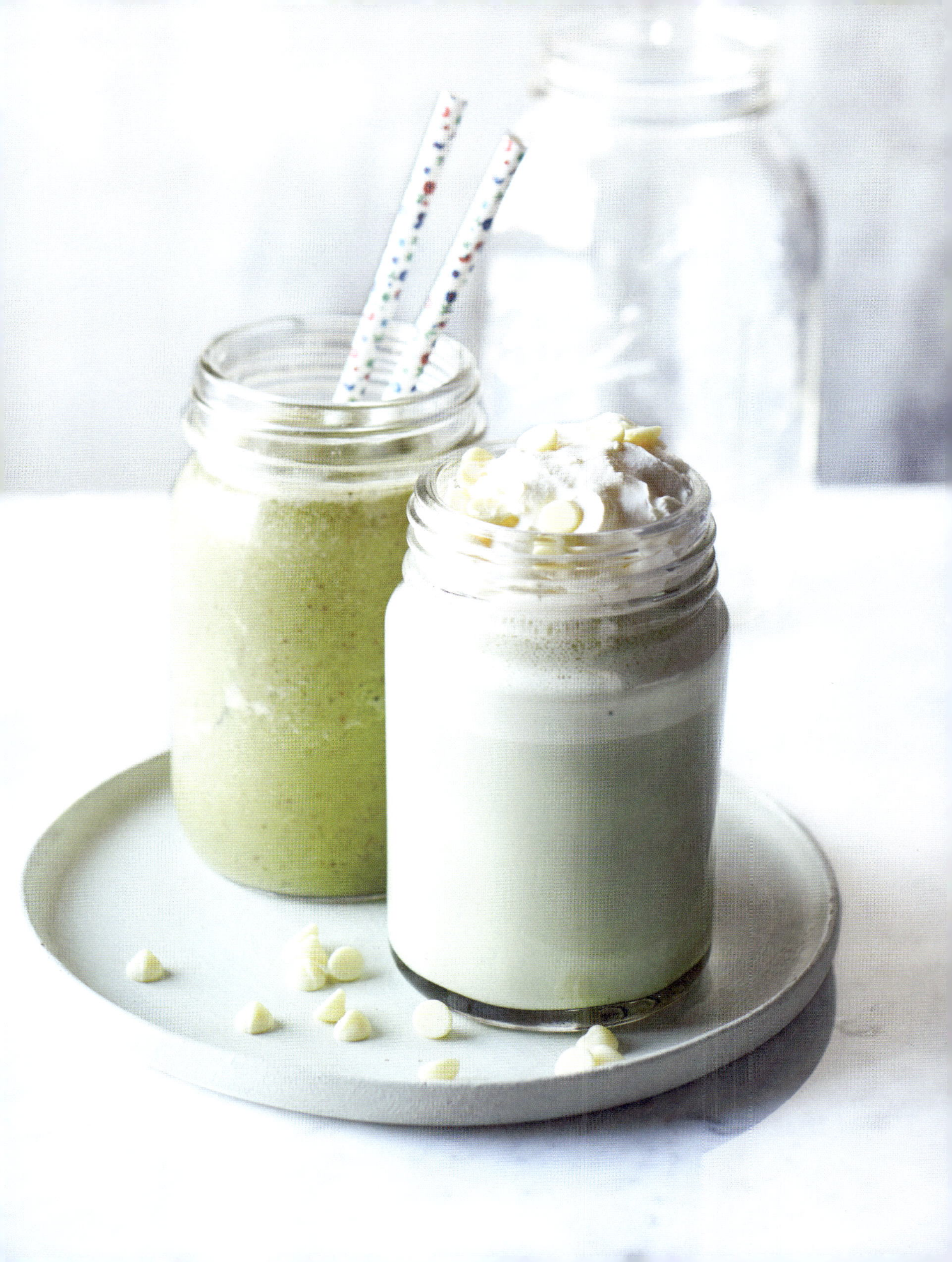

Matcha lemonade

This is one of our favourite lunchtime drinks and was created one hot summer's day in Brooklyn, New York. With lots of lemon, agave and matcha, this is a wonderfully zesty and fresh tonic.

SERVES 1

½ tsp matcha powder
squeeze of agave syrup
juice of 1 lemon
200ml (1 cup) sparkling (seltzer) water or soda water
handful of ice cubes, to serve
1–2 sprigs of mint, to serve

1 In a jug, mix the matcha powder and agave syrup into a paste.

2 Once dissolved, add the lemon juice and water.

3 Whisk well, then pour into a tall glass filled with ice, and serve with some mint leaves.

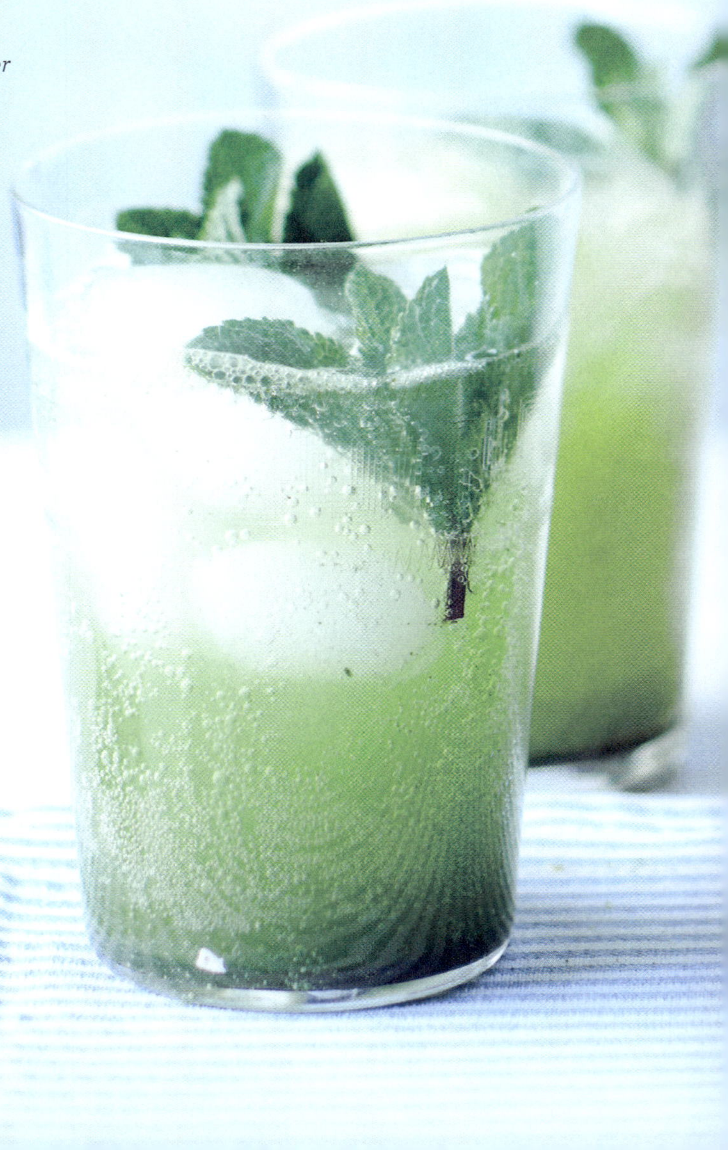

Matcha mint iced tea

This is a great green tea pick-me-up at the end of a long day. It's refreshing, sparkly and sophisticated – just add a splash of rum for a truly grown-up version.

SERVES 1

200ml (1 cup) sparkling (seltzer) or still water
½ tsp matcha powder
juice of 1 lime
handful of mint leaves
squeeze of runny honey
handful of ice cubes, to serve

1 Put the water, matcha powder, lime, mint and honey into a blender Blend until smooth.

2 Pour into a glass filled with ice and serve.

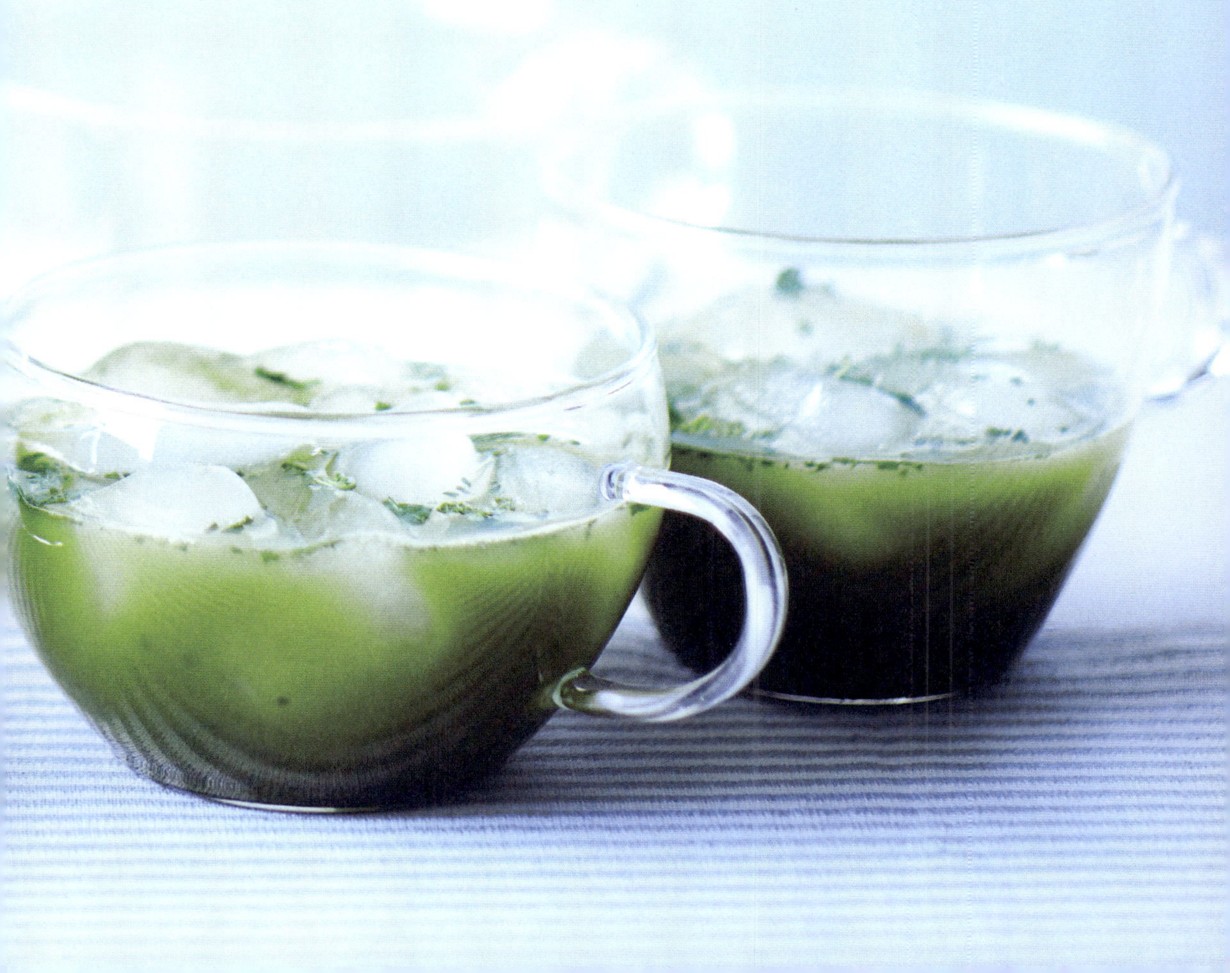

Matcha cocktails

With so many ways to bring a little green to cocktail hour, here are two inventive and incredibly tasty sips to awaken your inner mixologist.

Green martini

A vibrant twist on a classic and well-loved cocktail, the Grand Marnier complements the matcha perfectly in this elegant cocktail.

SERVES 1

½ tsp matcha powder
25ml (1½ tbsp) Grand Marnier
50ml (3 tbsp) vodka
4–5 ice cubes

1 Put all the ingredients into a cocktail shaker. Shake well then strain.

2 Pour into a martini glass and enjoy.

Mint fizz cocktail

Summer in a flute – this makes a great alternative to a classic Bellini or Kir Royale. Perfect for a celebratory drink, it packs a refreshing punch.

SERVES 1

6 mint leaves
½ tsp matcha powder
1 tsp agave syrup
juice of 1 lime
100ml (½ cup) chilled champagne

1 In a blender, pulverize the mint with the matcha powder, agave syrup and lime juice.

2 Pour in the champagne slowly. Stir gently until mixed well.

3 Pour into a champagne glass and serve chilled.

Citrus mocktail

Super tasty and slightly tart, to make this mocktail into a cocktail we suggest adding a measure of gin. Adults only!

SERVES 1

2 scoops of lemon sorbet
115ml (½ cup) ginger ale
4–5 mint leaves, chopped, plus extra to serve
juice of 1 lemon
½ tsp matcha powder

1 Place all the ingredients in a blender and blend until smooth.

2 Pour into a cocktail glass, garnish with mint leaves and serve.

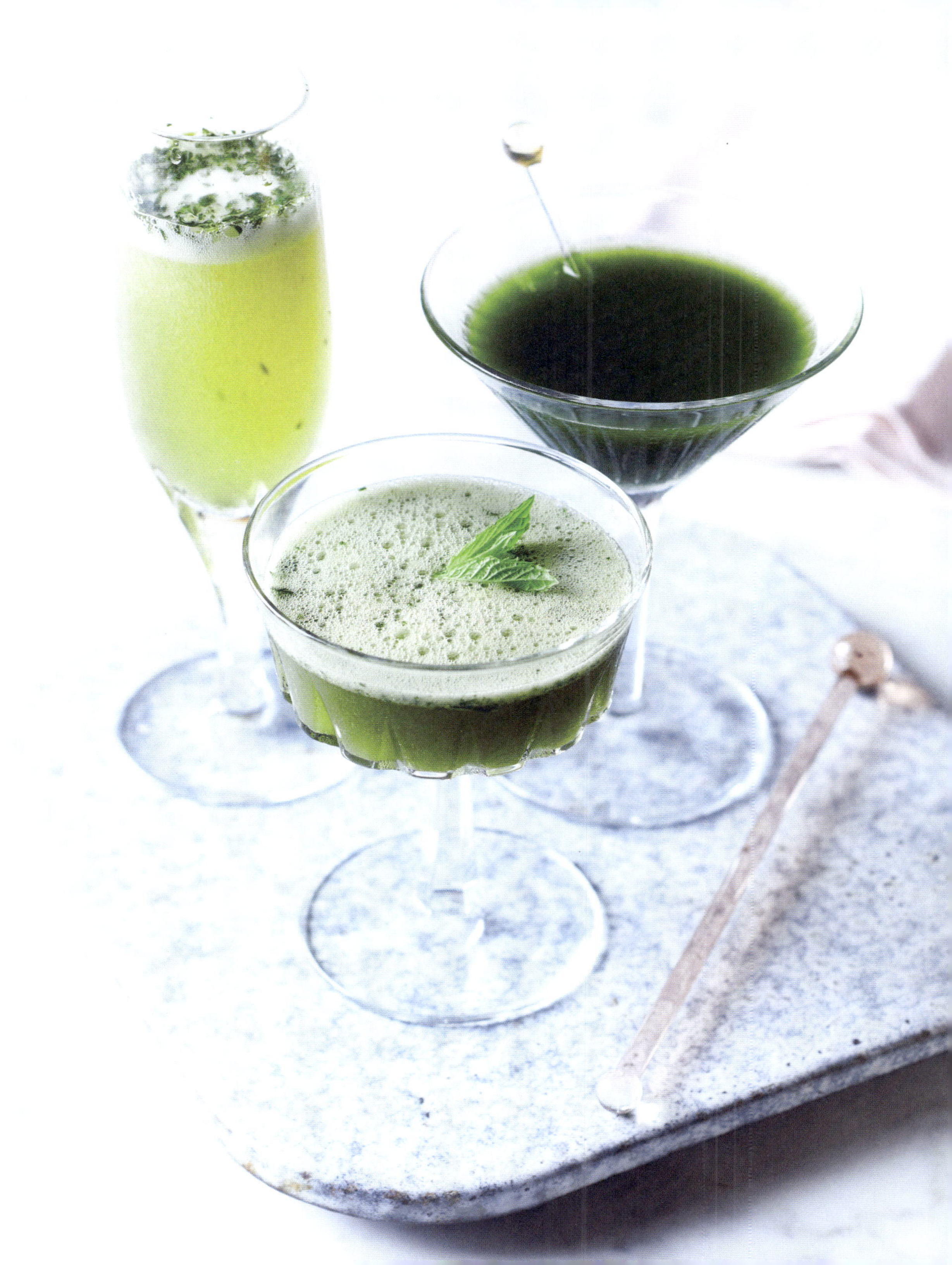

7

Breakfast

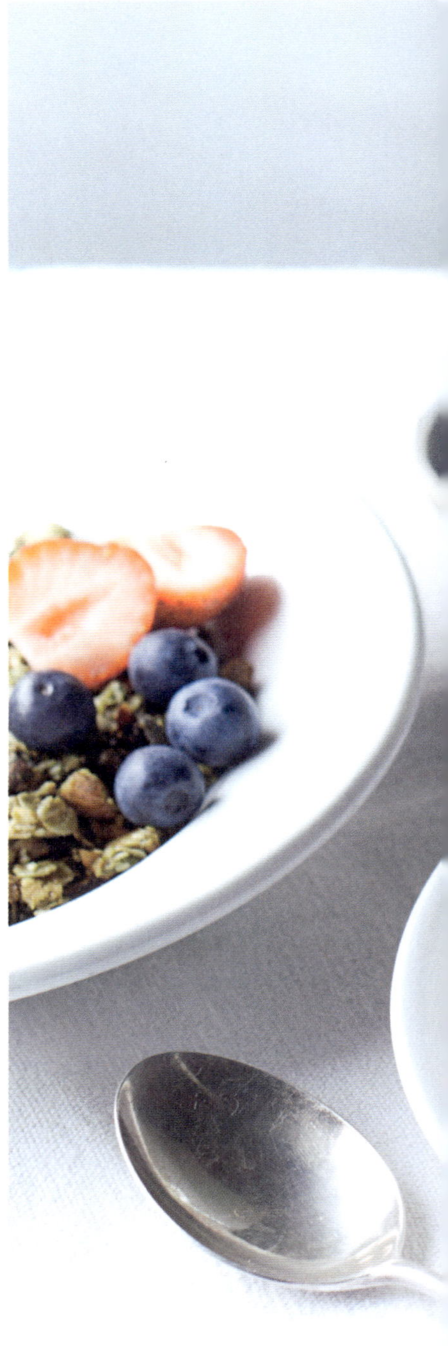

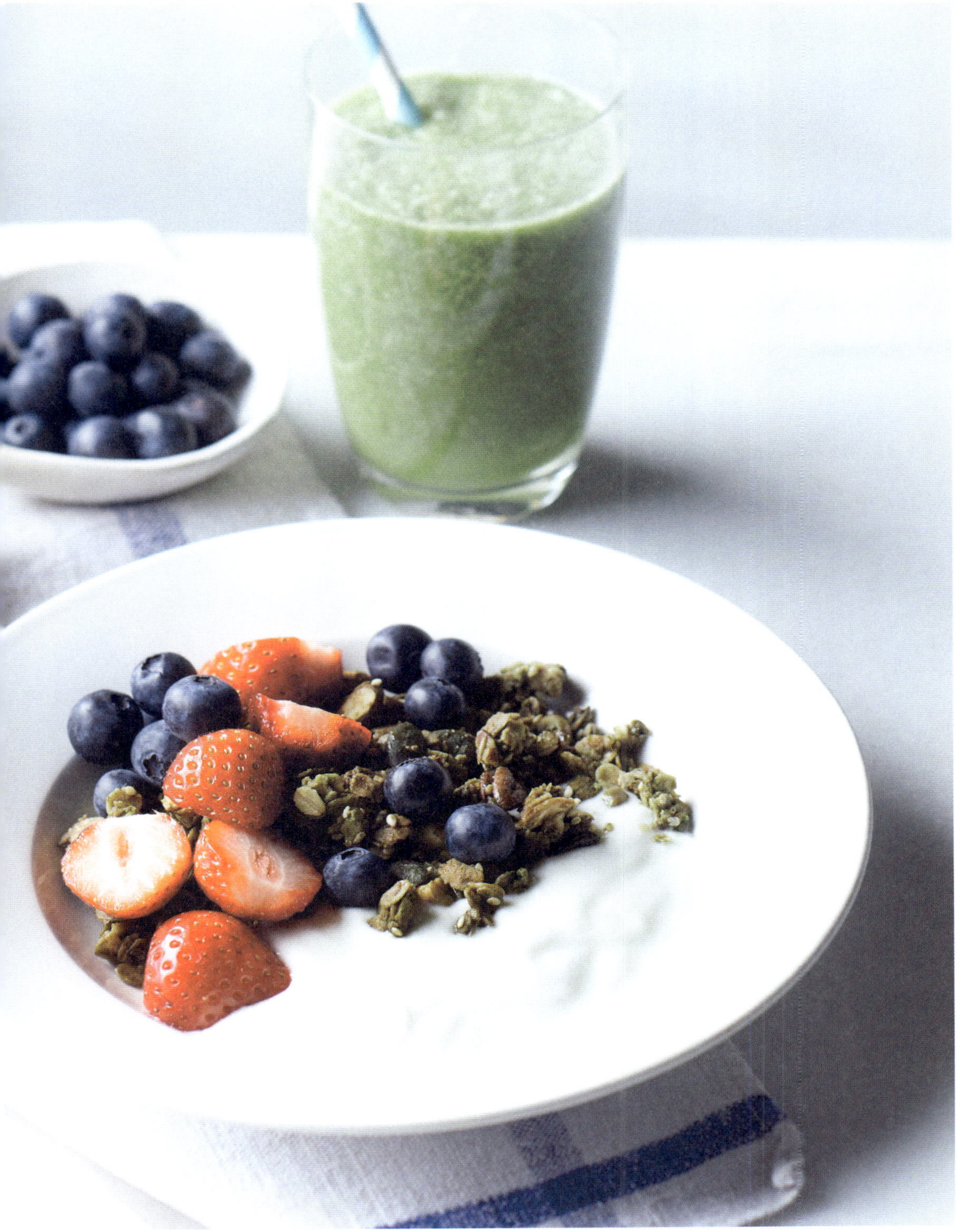

Matcha smoothies

Here are four delicious smoothies – great at any time of the day but especially at breakfast – with notes from Aidan and Glen that explain what makes them so healthy!

To make these nutritious smoothies, place all the ingredients in a blender (except the chocolate in the Hazelnut and vanilla smoothie) – adding the matcha last. Blend until smooth, pour into glasses and serve straight away.

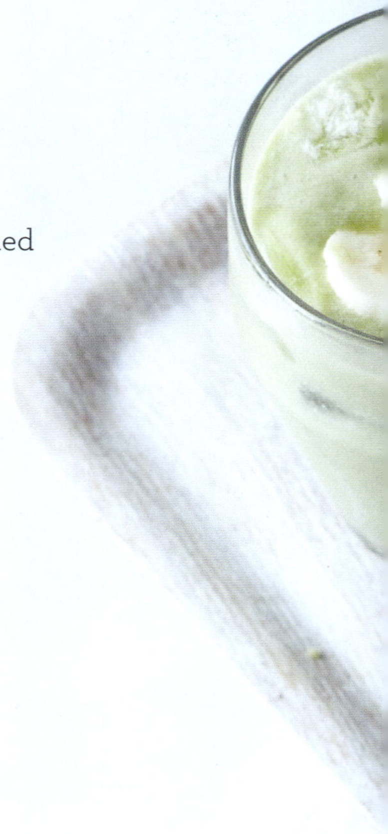

Hazelnut and vanilla smoothie

'Beauty in a glass. Bursting with skin-nourishing cocoa flavanols and omega-3, this smoothie is specially designed to make you beautiful from the inside out.'

SERVES 2

250ml (1¼ cups) hazelnut milk
2 tbsp natural yoghurt
6 strawberries, quartered
1 tsp flax seeds
½ tsp vanilla powder
1 tsp matcha powder
3 ice cubes (optional)

TO TOP
2 tsp dark (bittersweet) chocolate shavings (85% cocoa solids)

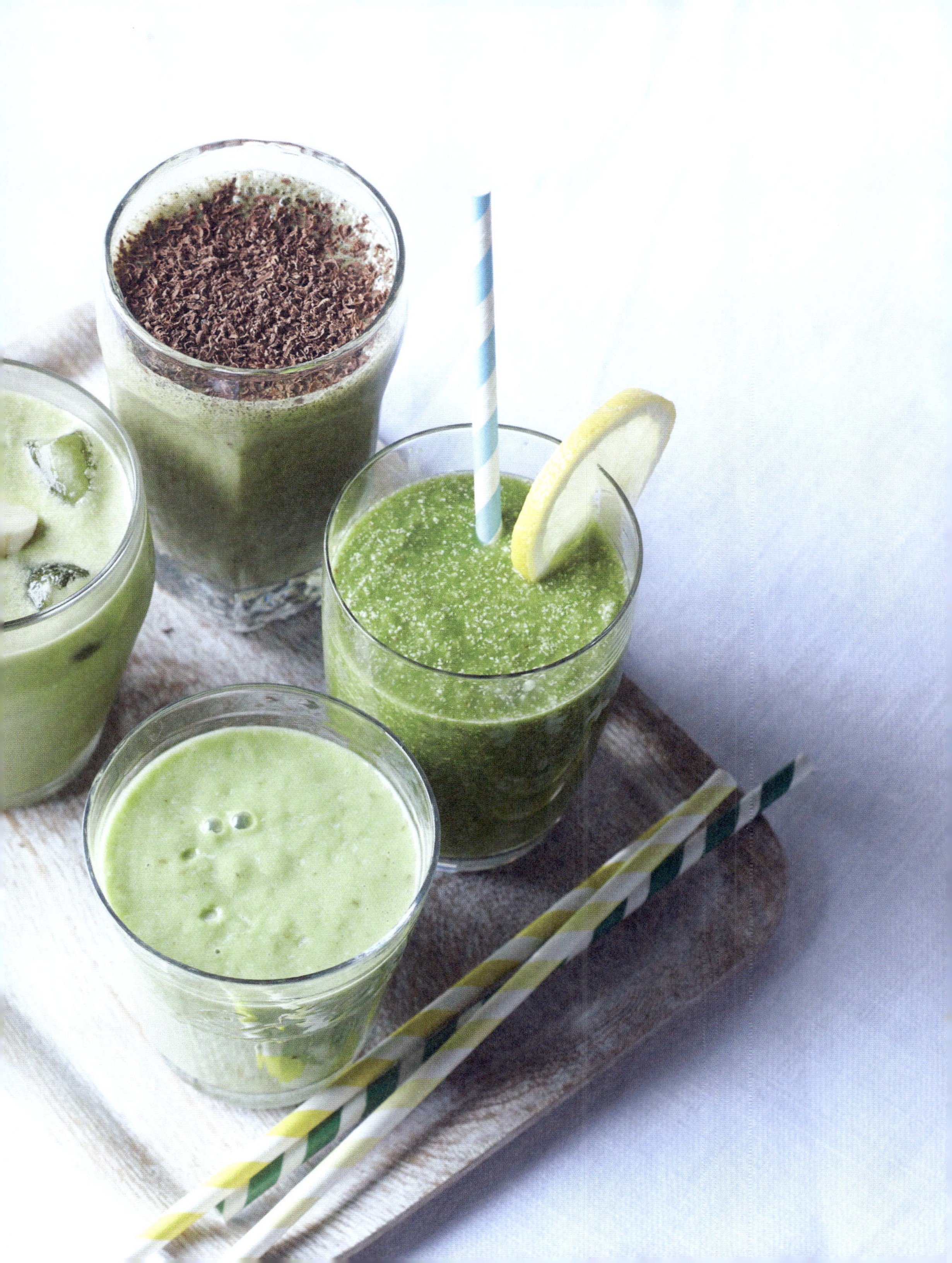

The green smoothie

'Experience matcha goodness in its ultimate form. The natural acids in the lemon juice help to enhance the absorption of EGCG. Best enjoyed on an empty stomach, this is a great smoothie to start any day.'

SERVES 2

25g (1oz) kale
10g (scant ½oz) rocket (arugula)
1 apple, cored and chopped
1 pear, cored and chopped
juice of 1 lemon
400ml (1¾ cups) coconut milk
1 tsp matcha powder
3 ice cubes (optional)

Dairy-free smoothie

'Creamy heaven – this smoothie is a delicious way to boost your intake of plant goodness! It's quick and easy to make your own fresh almond milk (see below), and almonds and matcha share many similar health benefits, making them a perfect pairing.'

SERVES 2

400ml (1¾ cups) unsweetened almond milk (see below)
3 dates, pitted and chopped
½ avocado
1 tsp matcha powder
3 ice cubes (optional)

HOMEMADE ALMOND MILK

Soak 145g (1 cup) blanched almonds overnight to soften them. In the morning, rinse well and blend in a high-powered blender with 500ml (2 cups) water.

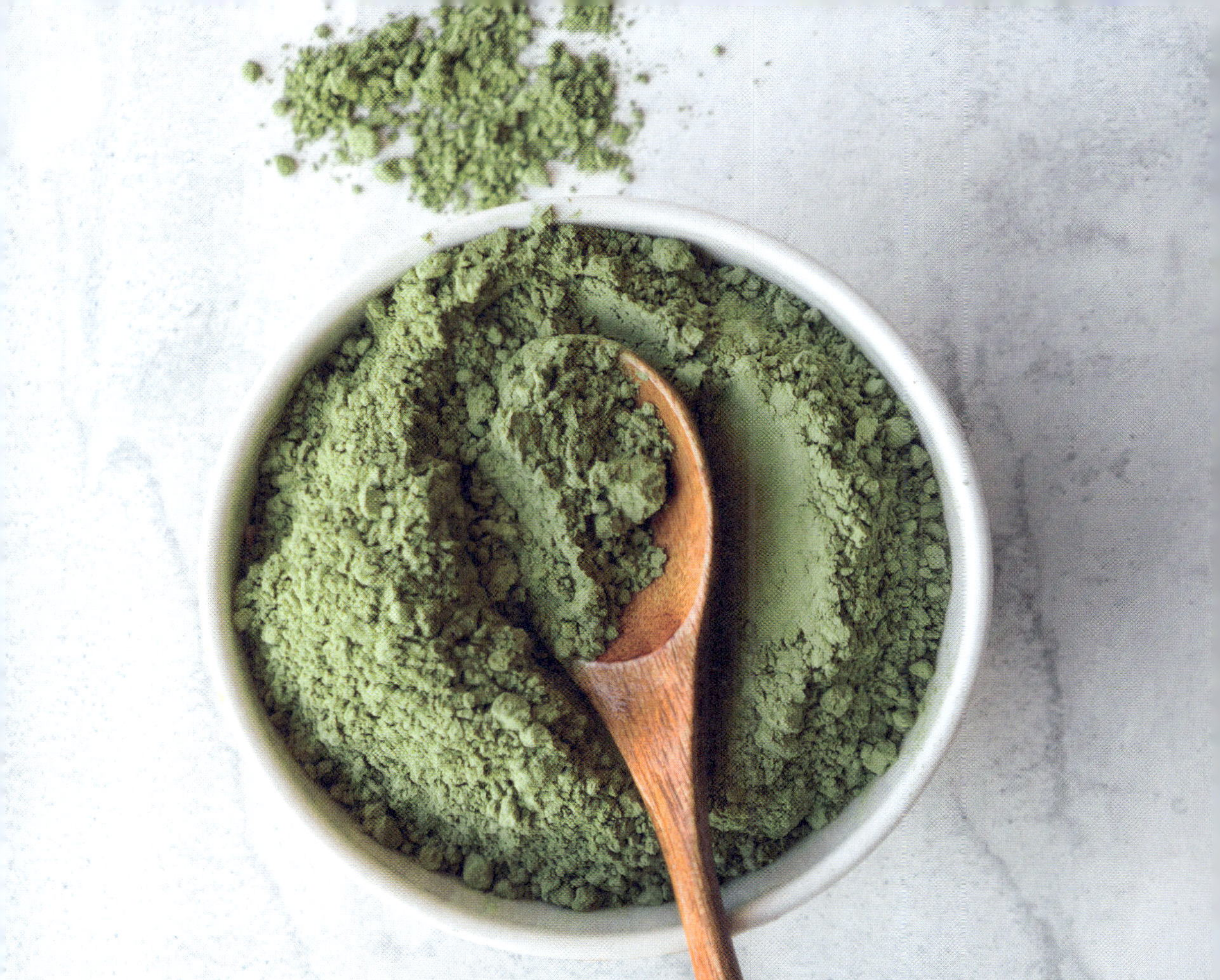

Coconut breakfast smoothie

Add some dark (bittersweet) chocolate shavings to the top of the smoothie, if you like, for a boost of cocoa flavanols.

SERVES 2

200ml (1 cup) coconut milk
2 tbsp coconut yoghurt
1 banana, sliced, plus extra to serve
1 tsp matcha powder

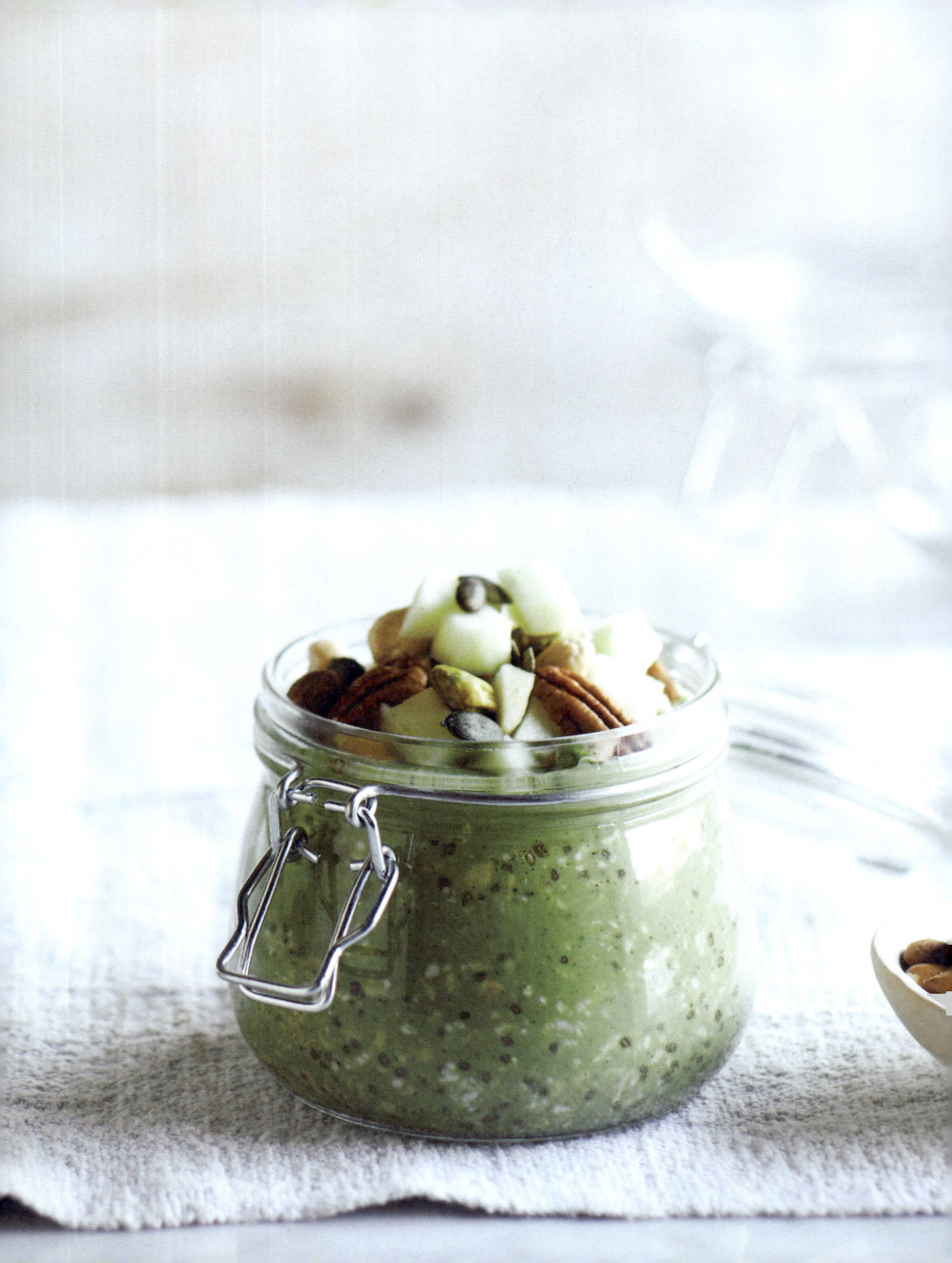

Matcha overnight oats

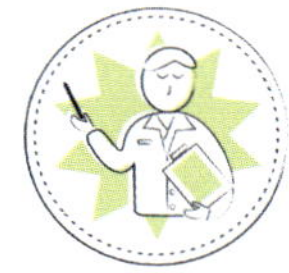

We worked with our nutritionists to devise this 'hearty' breakfast combining oats, apples, nuts and matcha – four key foods that they say 'help to lower cholesterol levels and slash the risk of heart disease.'

SERVES 2

FOR THE OATS

80g (1 cup) rolled oats
2 tsp chia seeds
375ml (1½ cups) almond milk (or hazelnut, rice or oat milk)
1 tsp matcha powder
2 pinches of ground cinnamon
1 tsp runny honey

FOR THE TOPPING

1 apple, peeled, cored and chopped
1 tsp pumpkin seeds
handful of mixed nuts

1 Prepare the oats in advance – ideally the night before you wish to eat them. Place the oats and chia seeds in a bowl or container.

2 In a separate bowl or jug, add 1 tbsp of the almond milk to the matcha powder and whisk with a hand-held whisk to make a smooth paste, then top with the rest of the milk. Mix until the matcha paste is fully blended into the almond milk.

3 Pour the matcha milk mixture over the oats, then stir in the cinnamon and honey. Cover and pop in the fridge overnight.

4 When ready to eat, transfer the oats to two bowls and top with the chopped apple, pumpkin seeds and nuts.

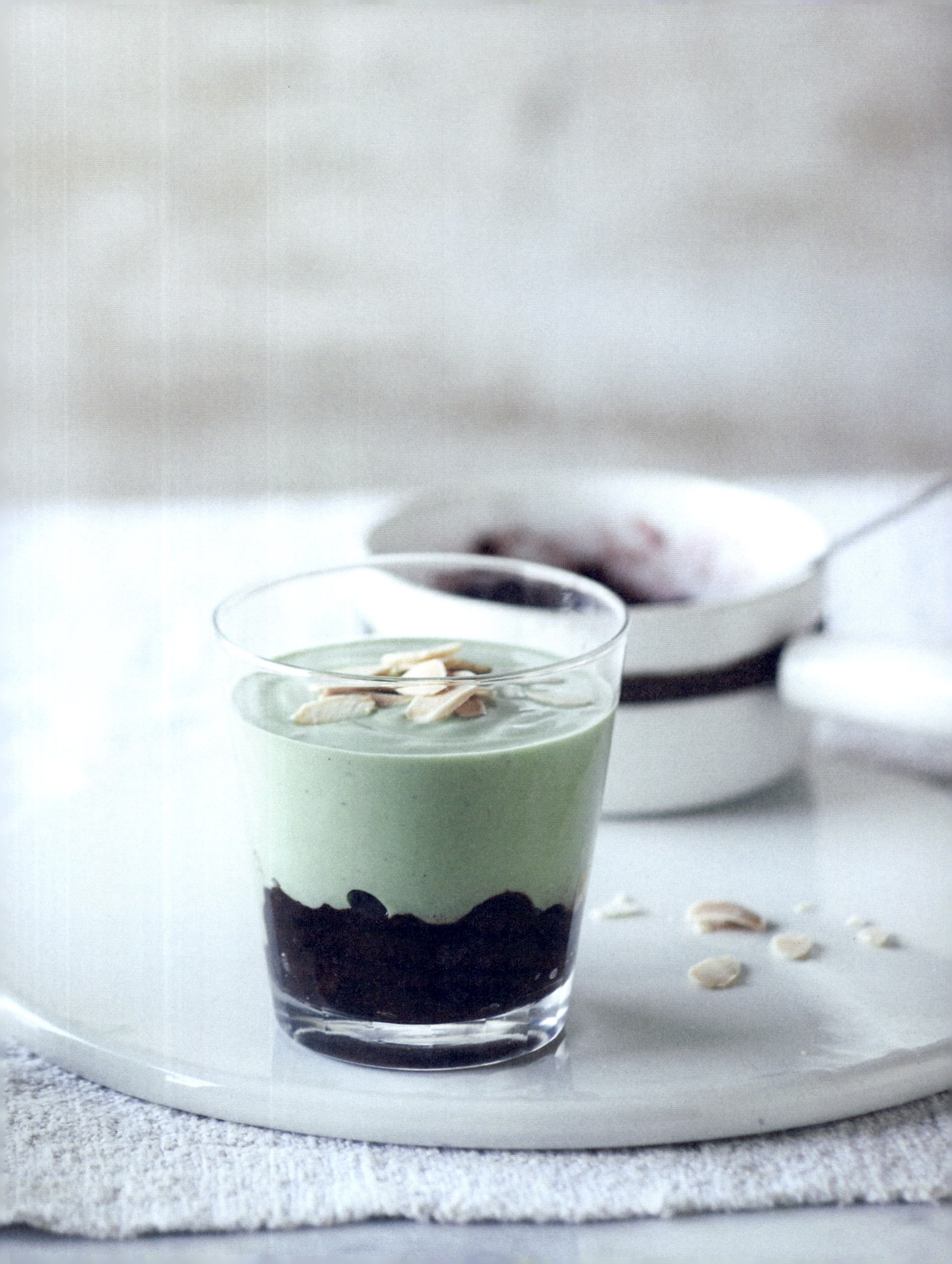

Matcha yoghurt with blueberry compote

'We're making no bones about it: this combo is designed to give your skeletal health a big boost. It's well known that we need sufficient calcium for healthy bones, and research now shows that natural plant compounds have dramatic benefit too, with berries, prunes and green tea being three leading contenders.'

SERVES 2

50g (½ cup) blueberries
4 prunes, chopped
1 tsp matcha powder
500ml (2 cups) natural yoghurt
1 tsp vanilla extract
handful of flaked almonds, to serve

1 To make the compote, place the blueberries and prunes in a small saucepan and cover with water (so the water just covers the fruit).

2 Bring to the boil then turn down to a simmer, stirring continuously until all the water has evaporated and you have a compote/jam consistency. Set aside to cool.

3 To make the matcha yoghurt, add the matcha powder to 2 tbsp of the yoghurt and whisk with a hand-held whisk to make a paste. Add the remaining yoghurt and the vanilla extract and stir well.

4 Once the compote is cool, transfer it into two glasses or bowls, top with the yogurt and flaked almonds and enjoy.

Matcha granola with berries

A fantastic breakfast for sustained energy as the oats provide 'slow-releasing' energy. Aidan and Glen have devised this recipe after exciting research has shown that natural compounds found in berries, green tea and cinnamon all have the ability to promote healthy blood sugar and insulin levels.

SERVES 4

2 tbsp coconut oil
100g (1 cup) rolled oats
80g (½ cup) mixed nuts, e.g. cashews, pistachios, almonds, pecans, chopped
1 tbsp pumpkin seeds
1 tbsp sesame seeds
1 tbsp matcha powder
½ tsp ground cinnamon
3 tbsp runny honey
400g (1¾ cups) Greek yoghurt
140g (1 cup) strawberries, halved or quartered
100g (⅔ cup) blueberries

1 Preheat the oven to 140°C fan/160°C/325°F/gas mark 3. Line a baking tray (sheet) with baking parchment.

2 To make the granola, heat the coconut oil gently in a saucepan until it melts. Remove from the heat and stir in the oats, nuts and seeds. Add the matcha powder, cinnamon and honey and mix together well.

3 Spread the granola mixture evenly over the lined baking tray and bake in the preheated oven for 15 minutes, turning it 2–3 times, until crisp and toasted.

4 Remove from the oven and cool thoroughly before storing in an airtight container.

5 To serve, layer the yoghurt, granola and berries in glass dishes, jars or pots.

VARIATIONS

- Experiment with other seasonal berries such as blackberries or redcurrants, or try dried cranberries, blueberries or goji berries.
- Add any of the following to the granola mix: sunflower and flax seeds, chopped dried figs or raisins, desiccated or dry shredded coconut, chopped Brazils or walnuts, or vanilla extract.
- This granola also tastes delicious with almond milk and fresh fruit.

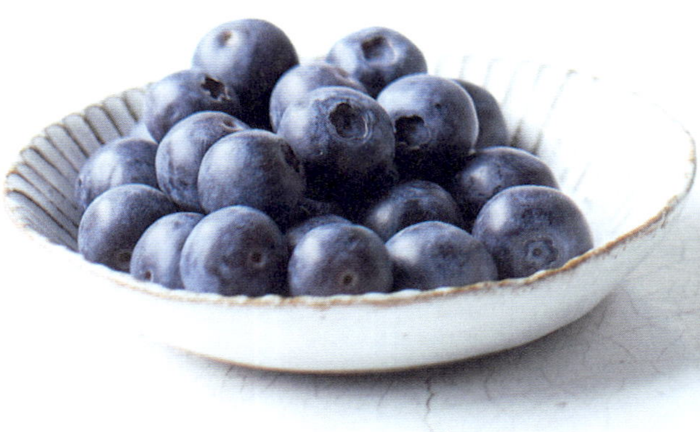

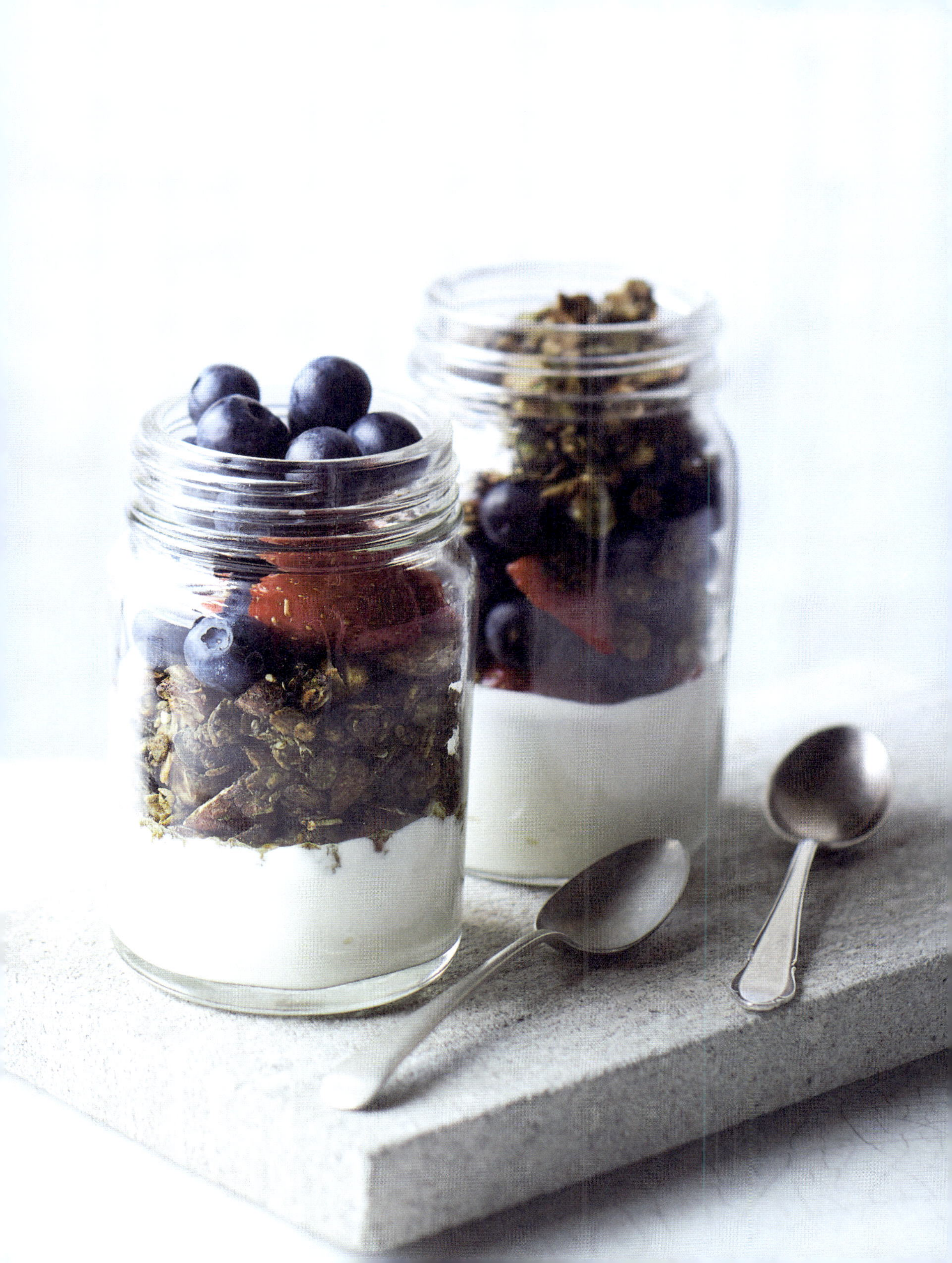

Matcha breakfast muffins

These muffins are hearty, oaty and very satisfying at breakfast. For a teatime version, add white or dark chocolate chips when you mix in the nuts, stirring them in gently.

MAKES 12 MUFFINS

100g (1 cup) rolled oats
200g (2 cups) plain (all-purpose) flour
2 tsp baking powder
1 tsp bicarbonate of (baking) soda
1 tbsp matcha powder
¼ tsp sea salt
85g (½ cup) light brown sugar
4 large ripe bananas
1 large egg, beaten
60g (½ cup) melted butter (or light olive oil)
85g (¾ cup) walnuts or pecans, chopped

1 Preheat the oven to 160°C fan/180°C/350°F/gas mark 4. Line a 12-hole muffin tin (pan) with paper baking cases (cupcake liners).

2 In a large bowl, combine the oats, flour, baking powder, bicarbonate of soda, matcha powder, salt and sugar. Mix together and make a well in the centre.

3 Mash the bananas with a fork in another bowl. Stir in the beaten egg and melted butter (or olive oil). Add to the dry mixture with the walnuts or pecans and fold through until just combined – take care not to over-mix. If the mixture seems too thick or a little dry, add a little orange juice or milk to thin it.

4 Spoon the mixture into the paper cases and bake in the preheated oven for 20–25 minutes until the muffins are well risen and a skewer inserted in the middle comes out clean.

5 Serve the muffins warm or cold. They can be kept fresh in an airtight container stored in a cool place for 2–3 days.

VARIATIONS

- You can flavour the muffins with a few drops of vanilla extract or add a little ground cinnamon, ginger and nutmeg for a spicy result.
- Mix in some freshly grated orange zest and the juice of 1 orange.
- For more fibre and texture, try stirring a tablespoon of flax seeds into the mixture. Or sprinkle the tops with pumpkin seeds before baking.

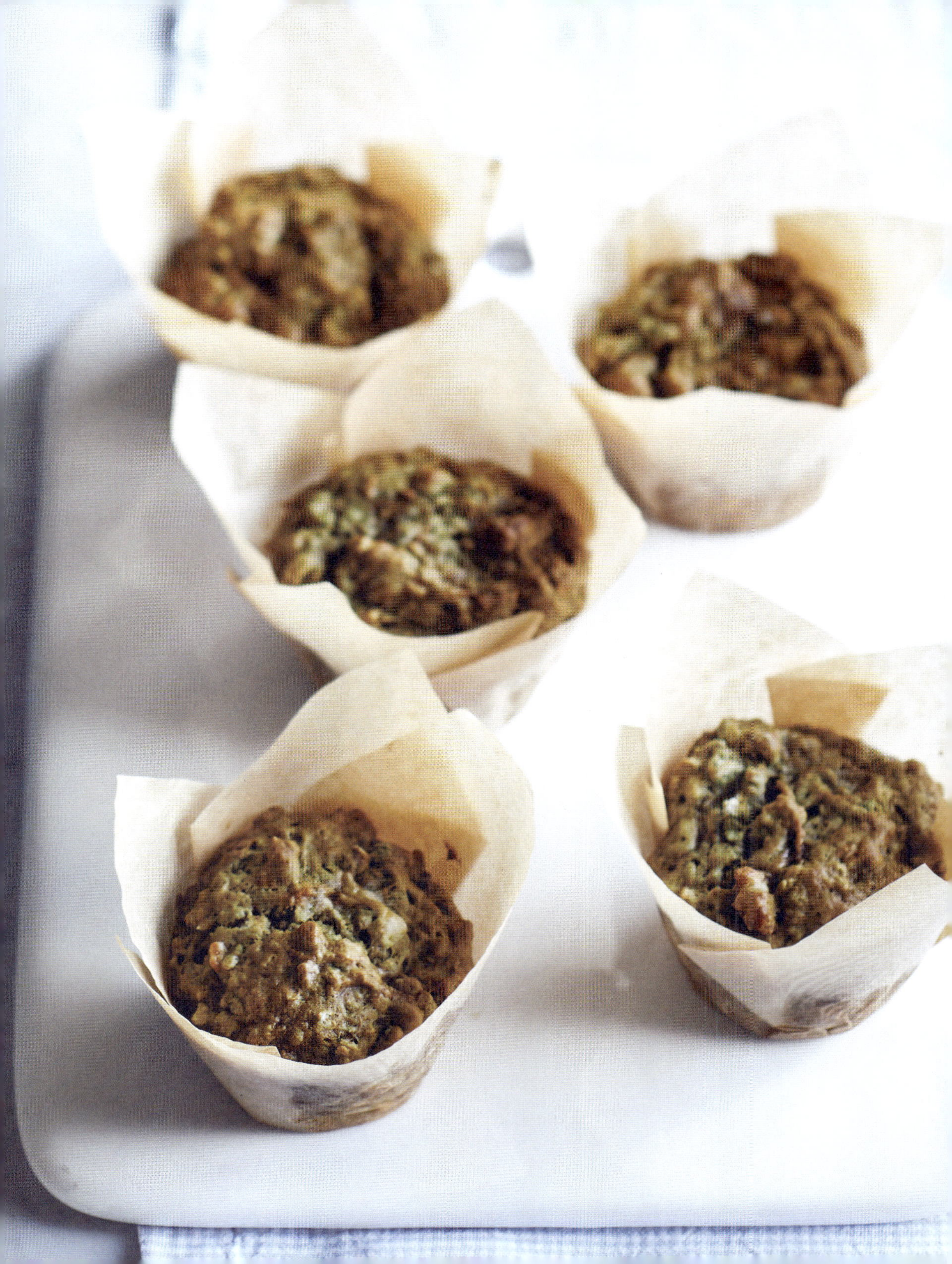

Matcha croissants

When we first heard you could get matcha croissants, we thought 'Wow!'. These look and taste amazing – deliciously buttery with a lovely, smooth matcha taste.

MAKES ABOUT 12 CROISSANTS

500g (5 cups) strong white bread flour, plus extra for dusting
1 tbsp matcha powder
2 tsp salt
60g (¼ cup) caster (superfine) sugar
14g (½oz) fast-action dried (instant) yeast
300ml (1¼ cups) cool water
300g (2½ sticks) unsalted butter, chilled
1 egg, beaten for glazing

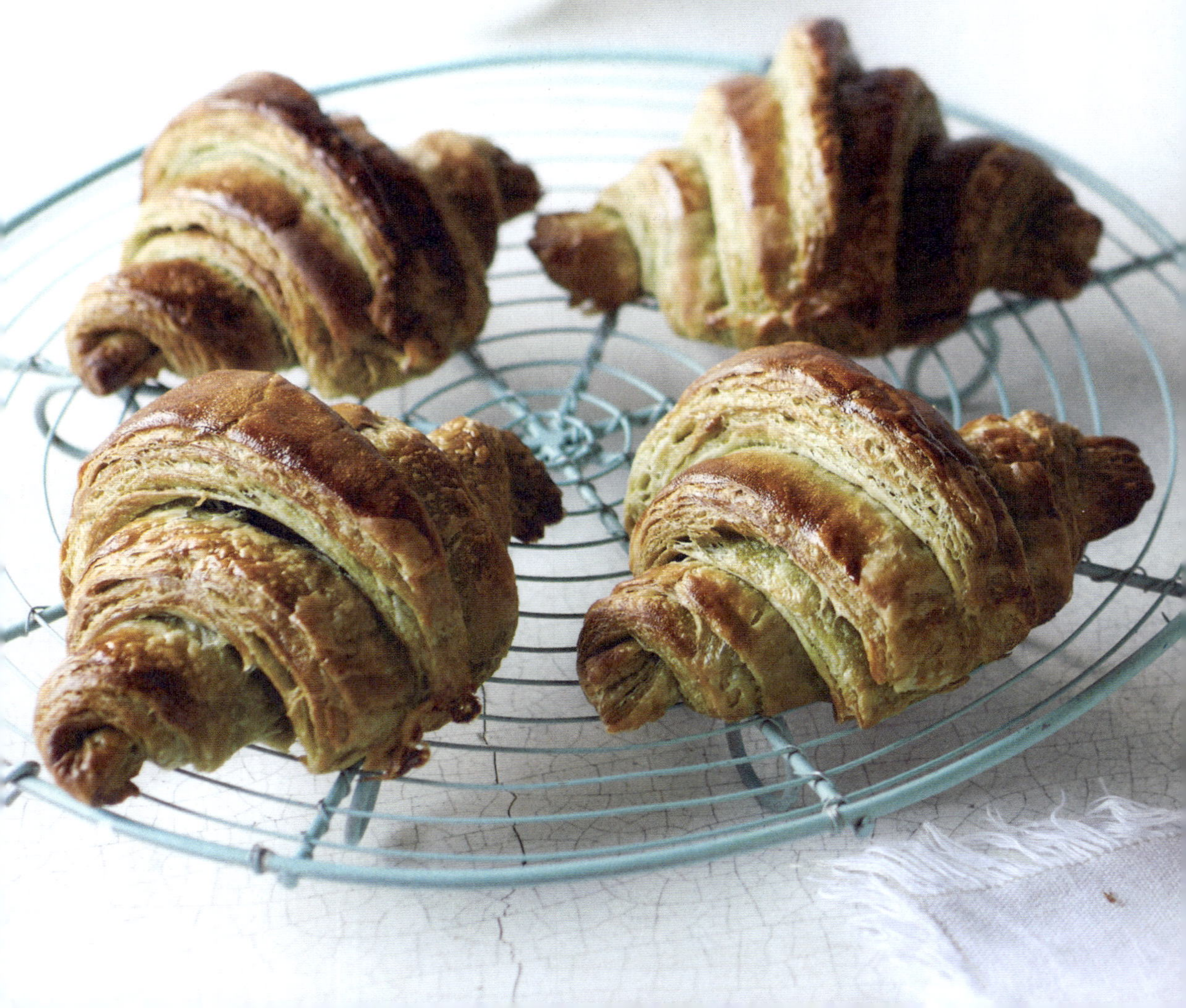

1. Put the flour, matcha powder, salt, sugar and yeast in a large mixing bowl. Make a well in the centre and gradually add the cool water, stirring well between additions.

2. When it's all added and mixed, take out the ball of dough and knead on a lightly floured work surface for about 10 minutes, until the dough is still quite stiff. Use the ball of your hand to push the dough away from you and stretch it before pulling it back and squashing it into a ball. Give it a quarter-turn, then repeat. Don't be gentle – really stretch and knead it hard to make it elastic. Alternatively, use a food (stand) mixer with a dough hook attachment.

3. Place the dough in a clean lightly oiled bowl and cover with cling film (plastic wrap) or in a plastic bag, and chill in the fridge for 1–2 hours.

4. Put the butter between 2 sheets of baking parchment and, using a rolling pin, bash it until you have a large rectangle, about 20 x 15cm (8 x 6in).

5. On a lightly floured surface, roll out the chilled dough to a large rectangle, about 40 x 20cm (16 x 8in). Place the butter in the centre of the dough and then fold the bottom third of the dough over to cover half of the butter. Next fold the top third of dough over to cover the remaining half of the butter.

6. Rotate the dough by a quarter turn and roll out slightly. Fold the short ends over to meet in the middle. Wrap in cling film and chill in the fridge for 30 minutes.

7. Repeat this rolling and folding process twice and then wrap and chill for at least 2 hours or, better still, overnight.

8. Line 2 baking trays (sheets) with baking parchment.

9. On a lightly floured surface, roll out the dough to a large rectangle, about 60 x 30cm (24 x 12in) and trim the edges. Cut the dough into 12 long triangles and gently stretch the corners at the base of each triangle to make it wider.

10. Starting at the wide base, gently roll up each triangle, working your way down to the point; tuck the point underneath. Bend the ends inwards and place on the prepared trays, leaving a little space between them.

11. Cover the trays with cling film and set aside for 2 hours at room temperature until the croissants double in size. Preheat the oven to 180°C fan/200°C/400°F/gas mark 6.

12. Brush the croissants generously with beaten egg and then bake in the preheated oven for 15–20 minutes until well risen and crisp. Cool on a wire rack before serving.

Matcha pancakes with maple syrup

Two of our favourite things – matcha and pancakes. Actually, matcha *in* pancakes. For a savoury brunch, serve the pancakes with crispy bacon rashers or grilled tomatoes and mushrooms.

SERVES 4

150g (1¼ cups) self-raising (rising) flour
1 tbsp matcha powder
2 tbsp caster (superfine) sugar
2 eggs
125ml (½ cup) semi-skimmed (skim) milk
2 tbsp butter, melted
sunflower or olive oil, for frying
maple syrup, to serve
blueberries, to serve

1 Preheat the oven on a very low setting – no more than 130°C fan/150°C/300°F/gas mark 2.

2 Sift the flour into a large bowl and mix in the matcha powder and sugar. Make a well in the centre.

3 In another bowl, whisk the eggs and then beat in the milk until well combined. Stir in the melted butter and pour into the well in the flour mixture. Whisk together until you have a smooth batter.

4 Place a large frying pan (skillet) over a medium heat and add a little oil. When it's hot, drop large spoonfuls of batter into the frying pan, leaving plenty of space between the pancakes. Cook for 1–2 minutes until golden underneath, then flip the pancakes over and cook the other side.

5 Remove to a plate and keep warm in the oven while you cook the remaining pancakes in the same way.

6 Divide the pancakes between four warm serving plates and serve immediately with maple syrup and a scattering of blueberries.

VARIATIONS

- Use buttermilk instead of semi-skimmed milk.
- Why not serve the pancakes with sliced banana or fresh raspberries or strawberries?
- Try adding a good pinch of cinnamon to the pancake mixture for a more subtle spicy flavour.

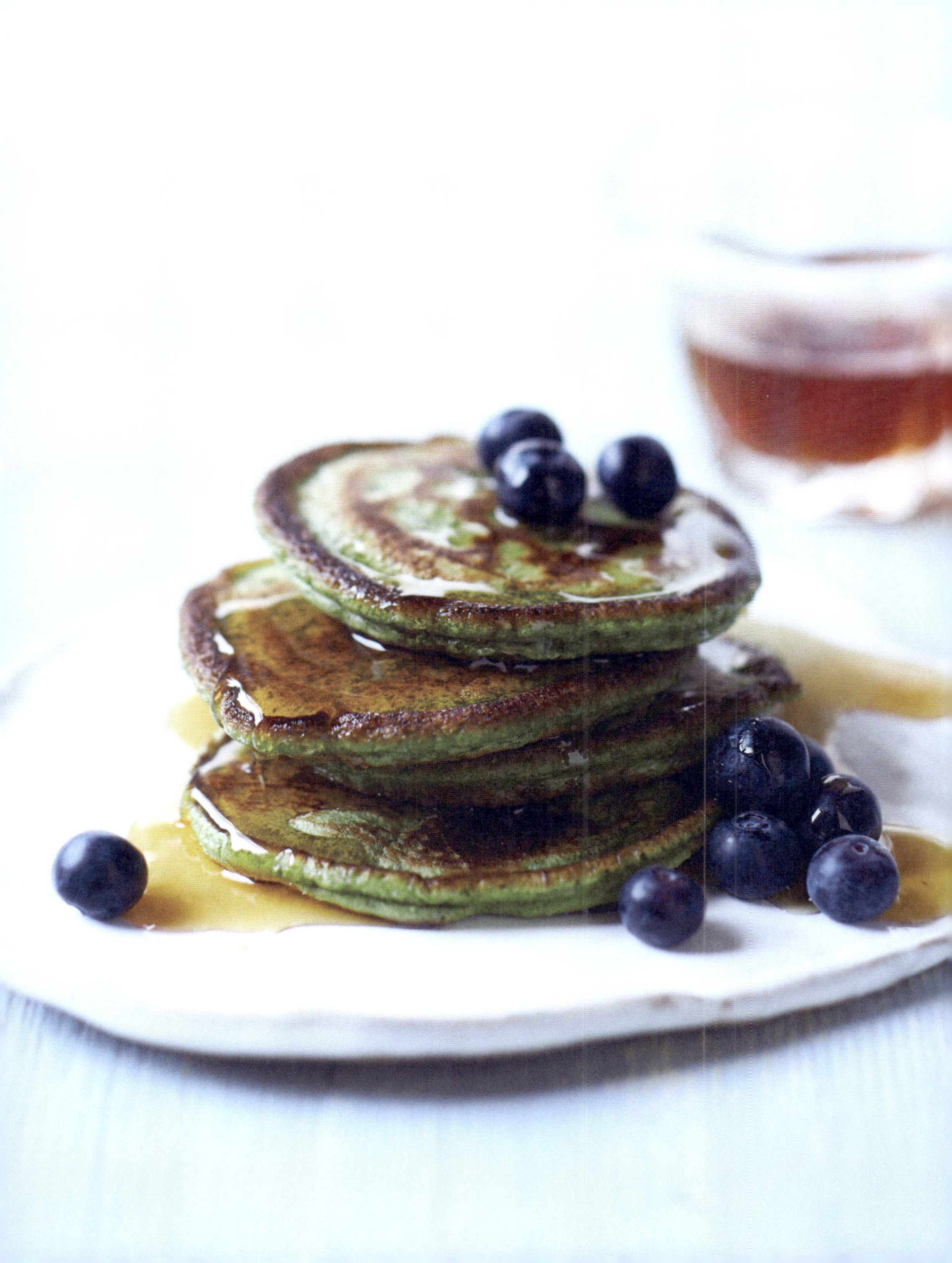

Matcha eggs Florentine

We admit this isn't the most obvious culinary combination, but trust us, it works. And we think it looks impressive, too! For matcha eggs Benedict, simply omit the spinach and top the eggs and hollandaise sauce with thin rashers of crispy lean back bacon.

SERVES 2

200g (7oz) baby spinach leaves
2 tsp white wine vinegar
4 eggs
2 English muffins, lightly toasted

FOR THE MATCHA HOLLANDAISE SAUCE
125g (1 stick) butter, diced
2 egg yolks
½ tbsp cold water
½ tbsp lemon juice
1 tsp matcha powder
salt and freshly ground black pepper

1 Make the hollandaise sauce: put the butter, egg yolks and water in a small saucepan over a low heat. Heat very gently, whisking continuously (use an electric one to make it easier), as the butter melts and the sauce starts to thicken. Turn up the heat a touch and keep on whisking until the sauce is thick enough to coat the back of a spoon. Gently stir in the lemon juice, matcha powder and seasoning to taste.

2 Remove the saucepan from the heat and cover with a lid to keep warm.

3 Meanwhile, put the spinach in another saucepan, cover with a lid and place over a very low heat for 2 minutes, until the spinach wilts and turns bright green. Drain in a colander and press down with a saucer to squeeze out all the liquid.

4 Heat a large saucepan of water until it's just simmering and add the vinegar. Carefully break the eggs into the saucepan and poach in the gently simmering water for about 4 minutes. When the whites are set and the yolks are still runny, remove with a slotted spoon and drain on kitchen paper (paper towels).

5 Place 2 toasted muffin halves on each serving plate and divide the spinach between them. Top each one with a poached egg and pour the hollandaise over the top. Serve immediately.

VARIATIONS

- If you're in a hurry, top the eggs with some shop-bought hollandaise sauce and sprinkle with a pinch of vivid green matcha sea salt. Just grind together equal parts of matcha powder and coarse sea salt crystals in a pestle and mortar.
- Substitute thinly sliced smoked salmon or tuna mayo for the spinach.

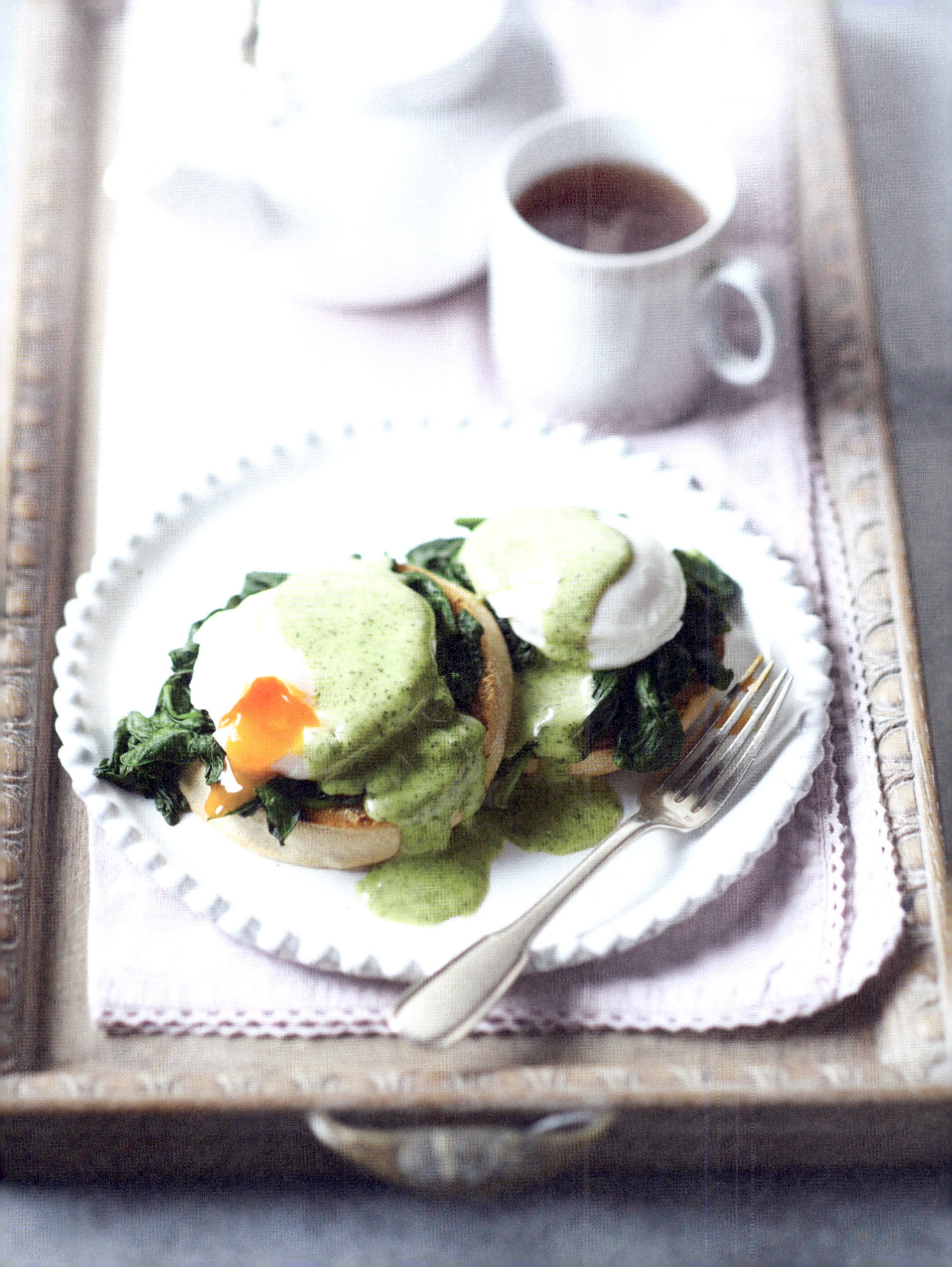

Snacks

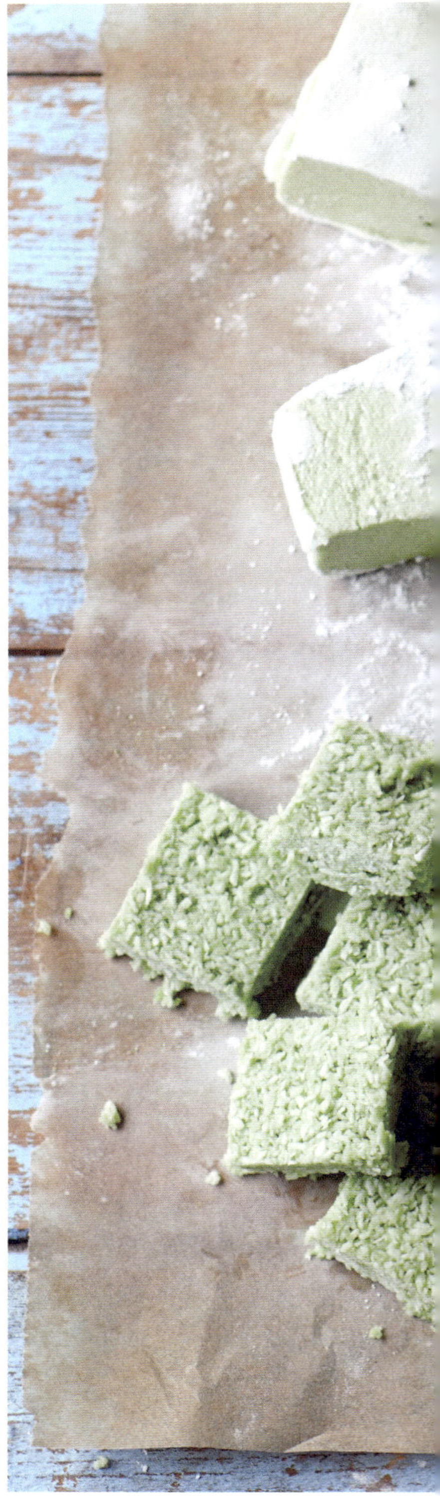

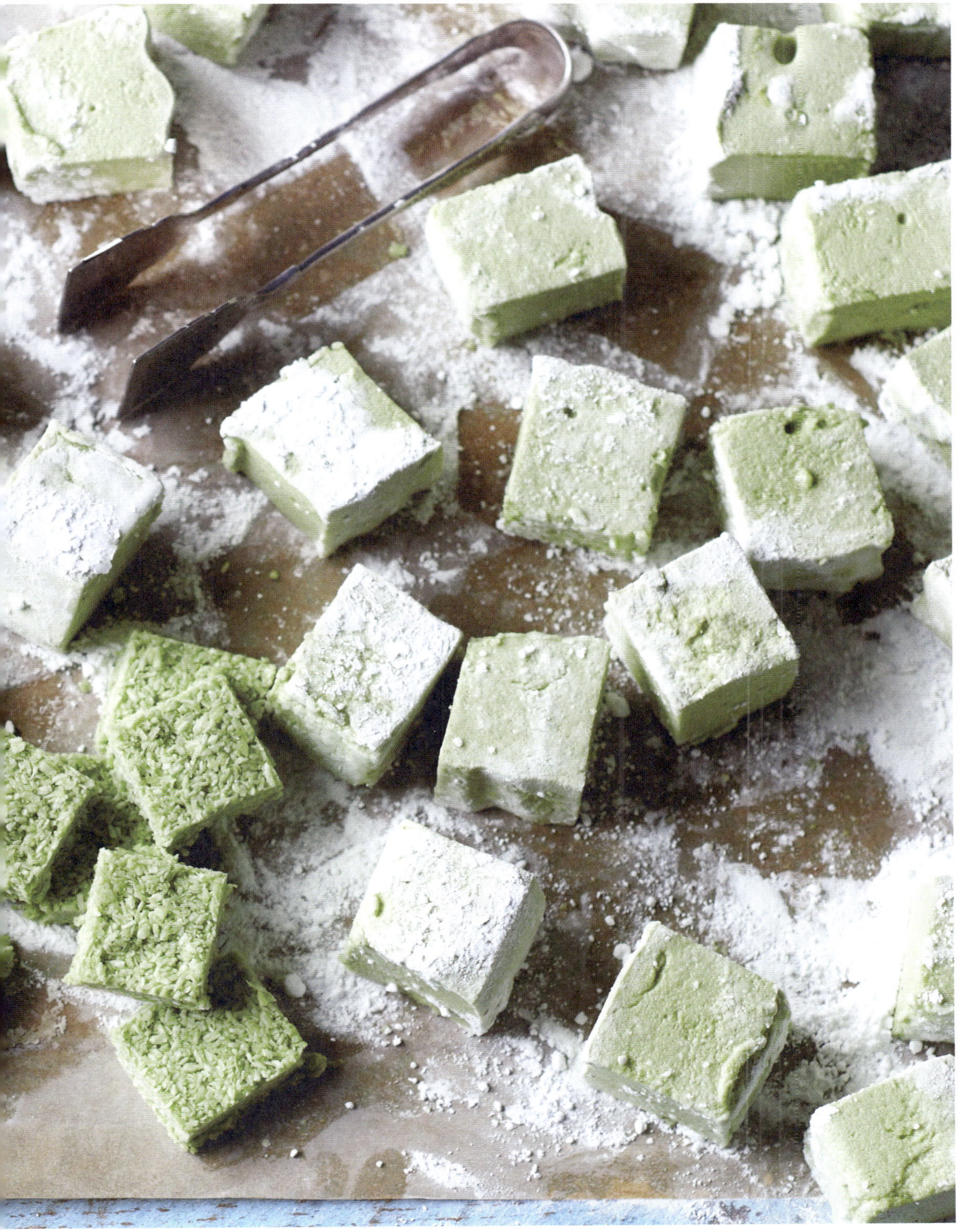

Chia seed and matcha power pots

You need to make these the night before you want to enjoy them. It's well worth doing though, as Aidan and Glen believe these are 'a real humdinger of a snack, packed full of healthy fats and protein from nuts and seeds. Designed to keep hunger at bay, these power pots provide slow-burn fuel to comfortably see you through the longest of mornings or afternoons.'

SERVES 4

8 tbsp chia seeds
500ml (2 cups) unsweetened almond milk
2 tsp matcha powder
1 tbsp runny honey or date syrup
2 ripe peaches, stoned (pitted) and diced
4 tbsp Greek yoghurt
150g (1½ cups) blueberries
4 tbsp mixed nuts, e.g. almonds, hazelnuts or pistachios, chopped

1 Put the chia seeds and almond milk in a bowl and stir together.

2 In another bowl, blend the matcha powder and honey or date syrup until evenly mixed, then stir into the chia mixture with the diced peaches.

3 Divide the mixture between four bowls, glass pots or screwtop jam jars and cover with cling film (plastic wrap) or the screwtop lids.

4 Chill in the fridge overnight or until all the liquid is absorbed and the mixture has a jelly-like texture.

5 The following day, top each pot with a spoonful of yoghurt and then sprinkle with the blueberries and chopped nuts.

VARIATIONS

- Experiment with different fruit, depending on what's in season. Try diced apple or pear, strawberries, raspberries, cherries or plums.
- Instead of fresh fruit, top with fruit compote before adding the yoghurt.
- Spoon a layer of mango purée into the bottom of each pot before adding the chia mixture for a colourful layered effect.

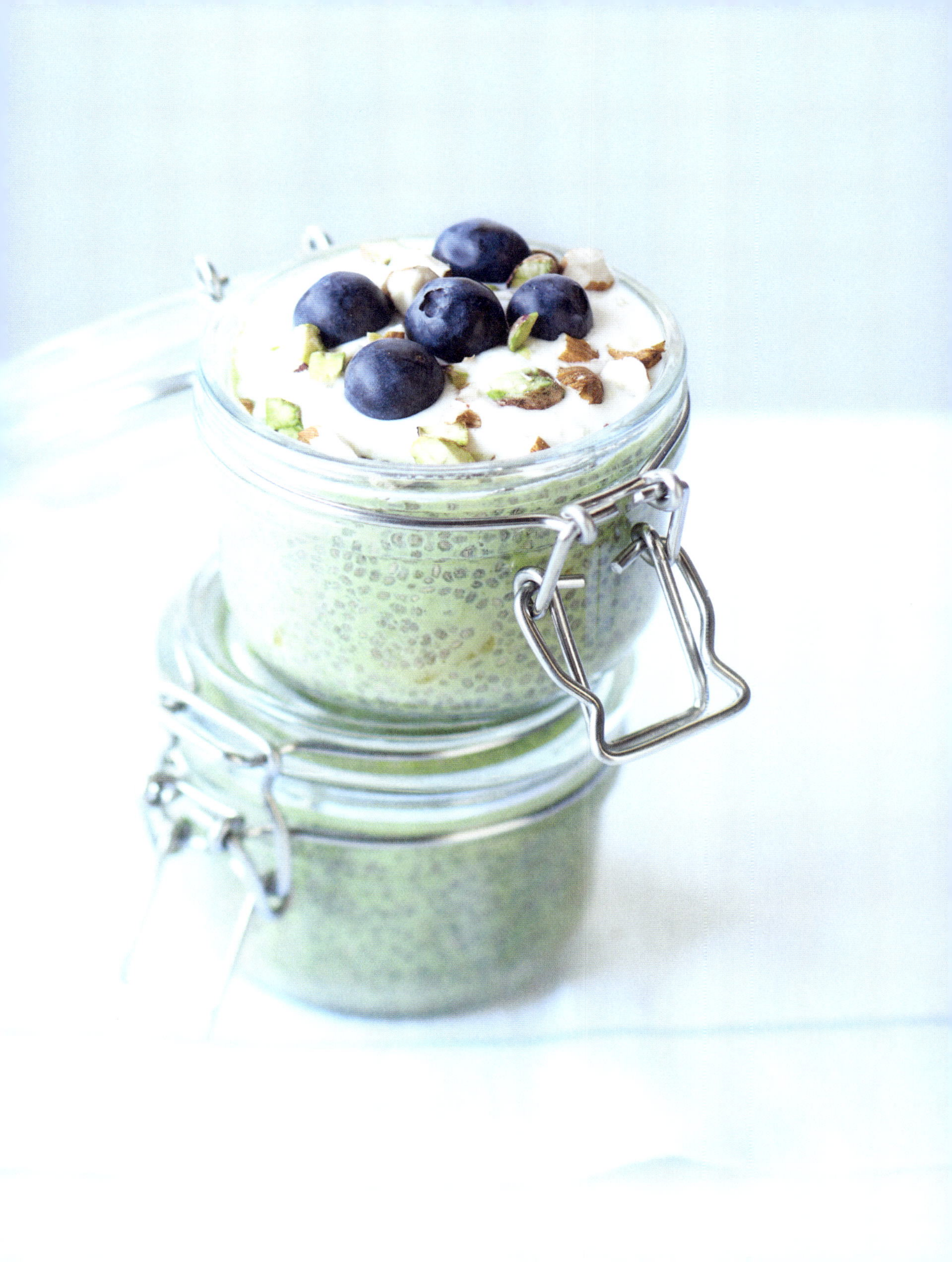

Matcha pretzels

Matcha works really well with soft, sweet breads and pretzels, and we love this pretzel recipe with its distinctive 'sweet and salty' taste.

MAKES 10–12 PRETZELS

450g (4½ cups) strong white bread flour, plus extra for dusting
7g (¼oz) fast-action dried (instant) yeast
1 tsp salt
1 tbsp soft brown sugar
3 tbsp bicarbonate of (baking) soda
1 tbsp matcha powder
125ml (½ cup) warm water
125ml (½ cup) milk
2 tbsp butter, at room temperature
1 egg, beaten
sea salt crystals and toasted sesame seeds

1 Put the flour, yeast, salt, sugar and 1 tablespoon of the bicarbonate of soda in a large mixing bowl and mix together. Make a well in the centre.

2 Whisk the matcha powder into the warm water until it is smooth and free of lumps. Pour into the flour mixture with the milk and add the softened butter. Mix together until you have a soft, smooth dough.

3 Turn the dough out onto a lightly floured surface and knead well for 5–10 minutes until it becomes elastic, silky in texture and doesn't stick to your fingers.

4 Place the dough in a lightly oiled clean bowl, then cover and set aside for 1–2 hours until it has doubled in size. There's no need to put it in a warm place – leave it at room temperature.

5 Knock the dough back and knead briefly, then cut it into 10–12 equal-sized pieces. Using your hands, stretch each piece out and roll into a sausage shape with the ends slightly slimmer than the middle. Cross the ends over each other and then fold them up and over into the centre of the loop to make a classic pretzel shape (see the photograph opposite). Leave them for 30 minutes to rise and puff up a little.

6 Preheat the oven to 180°C fan/200°C/400°F/gas mark 6. Line 2 baking trays (sheets) with baking parchment.

7 Bring a large saucepan of water to the boil and add the remaining bicarbonate of soda. Add the pretzels, a few at a time, and boil for 20 seconds. Remove with a slotted spoon and place on the baking trays. Brush with beaten egg and then sprinkle with sea salt and sesame seeds.

8 Bake in the preheated oven for 12–15 minutes until golden brown and firm. Allow to cool and store in an airtight container.

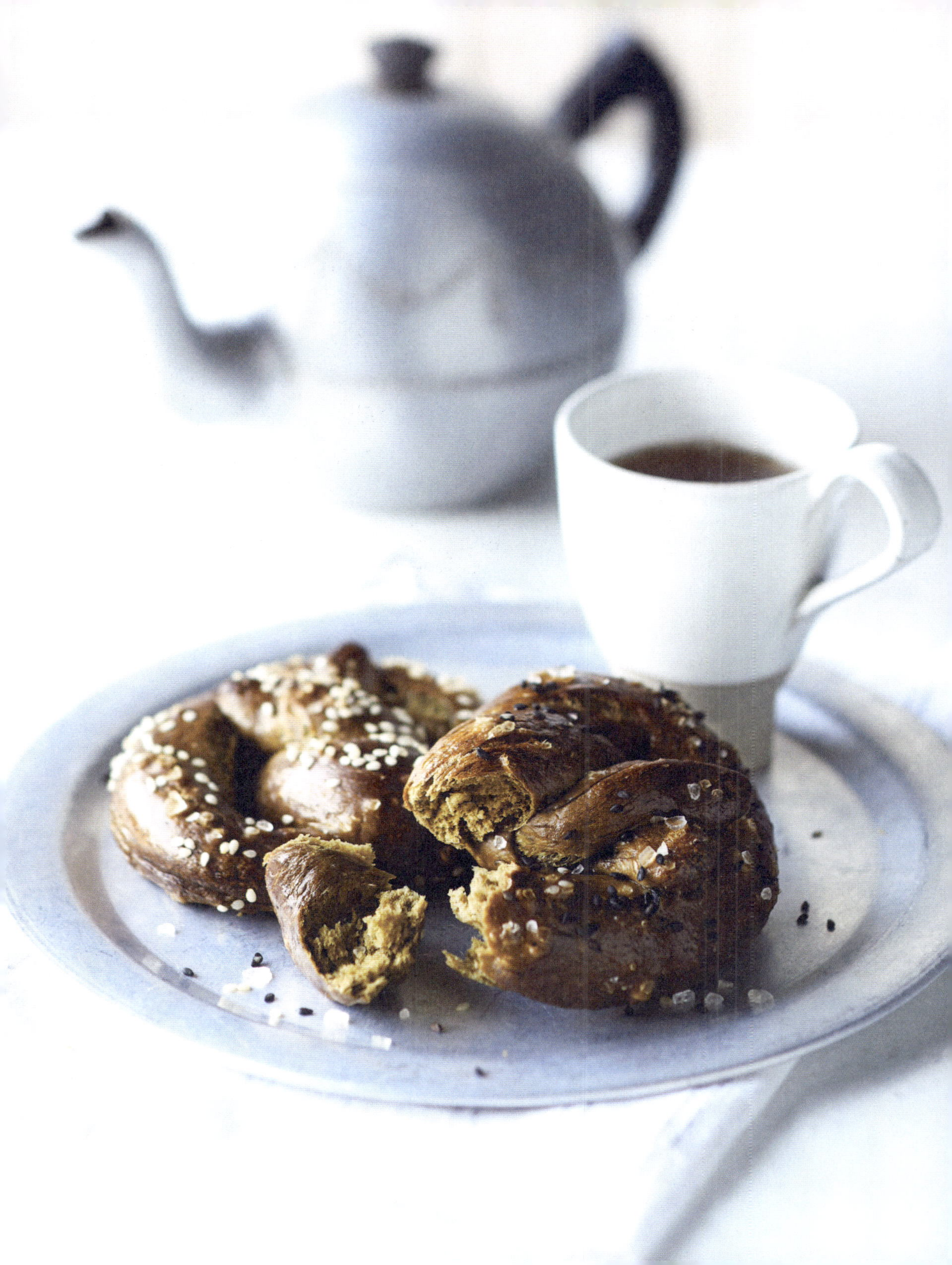

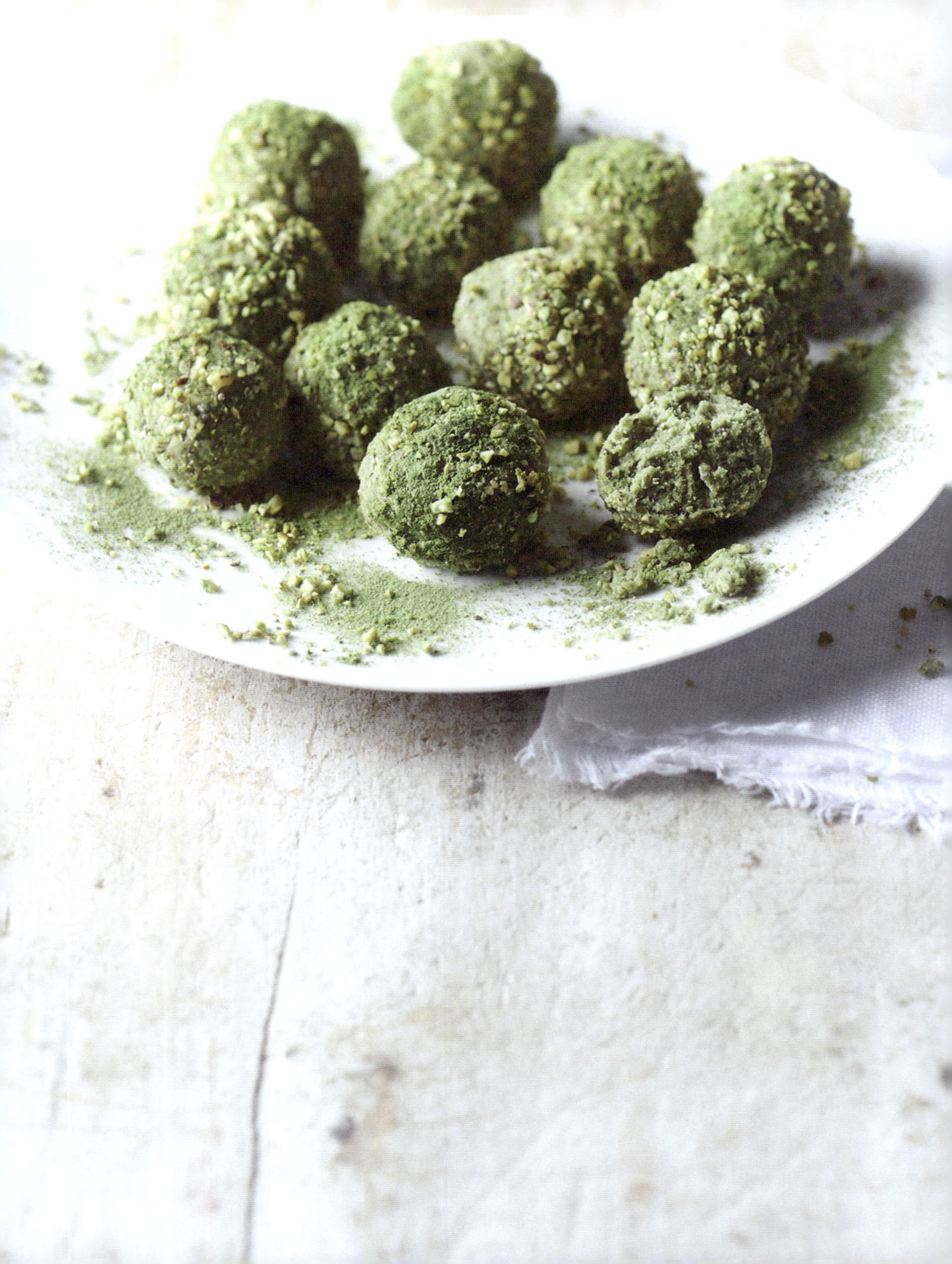

Matcha pistachio protein balls

'These are a superb pick-me-up for anyone keeping active. Add your favourite dried fruits, such as chopped dates, apricots or figs, or even some raw cacao.'

MAKES 12 BALLS

75g (½ cup) cashews
40g (½ cup) unsweetened desiccated coconut
1 tbsp chia seeds
2 tsp matcha powder, plus extra for rolling
2 tbsp coconut flour
30g (¼ cup) protein powder
2 tbsp coconut oil
4 tbsp runny honey or date syrup
3–4 tbsp water
30g (¼ cup) pistachio nuts, finely chopped

1 In a food processor or blender, blitz the cashews, coconut, chia seeds, matcha powder, coconut flour and protein powder.

2 Melt the coconut oil in a small saucepan over a low heat and add to the blended mixture with the honey and the water. Blitz briefly until you have a dough. Add a little more water if it's too dry – you want it to stick together.

3 Divide the mixture into 12 equal-sized portions and, using your hands, roll each one into a ball.

4 Roll the balls in the pistachios and some matcha powder, then chill in the fridge until cool and firm. You can store them in the fridge in an airtight container.

Raw sticky date and matcha bars

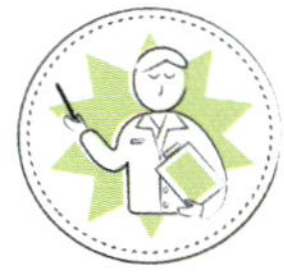

'These bars are proof that guiltless pleasure does exist. Medjool dates are a fantastic sweet treat that actually improve health and blood sugar levels.'

MAKES 8–10 BARS

2 tbsp coconut oil, plus extra for greasing
175g (1 cup) medjool dates, pitted
75g (½ cup) almonds
1 tbsp matcha powder
30g (½ cup) flax seeds
1 tsp vanilla extract
75g (¾ cup) rolled oats
coconut flakes and matcha powder, for sprinkling

1 Lightly grease a small square or rectangular tin (pan) or baking dish with a little coconut oil and then line with baking parchment. Melt the coconut oil in a small saucepan over a low heat.

2 Blitz the dates, almonds, matcha powder, flax seeds, vanilla extract and melted coconut oil to a purée in a food processor. Stir in the oats. If the mixture is too loose and sticky, add more oats.

3 Spoon the mixture into the lined tin, pushing it right into the corners and pressing it down evenly. Sprinkle with coconut flakes and matcha and level the top, pressing down with a spatula or spoon.

4 Chill in the fridge until set. Cut into bars and store in an airtight container in the fridge.

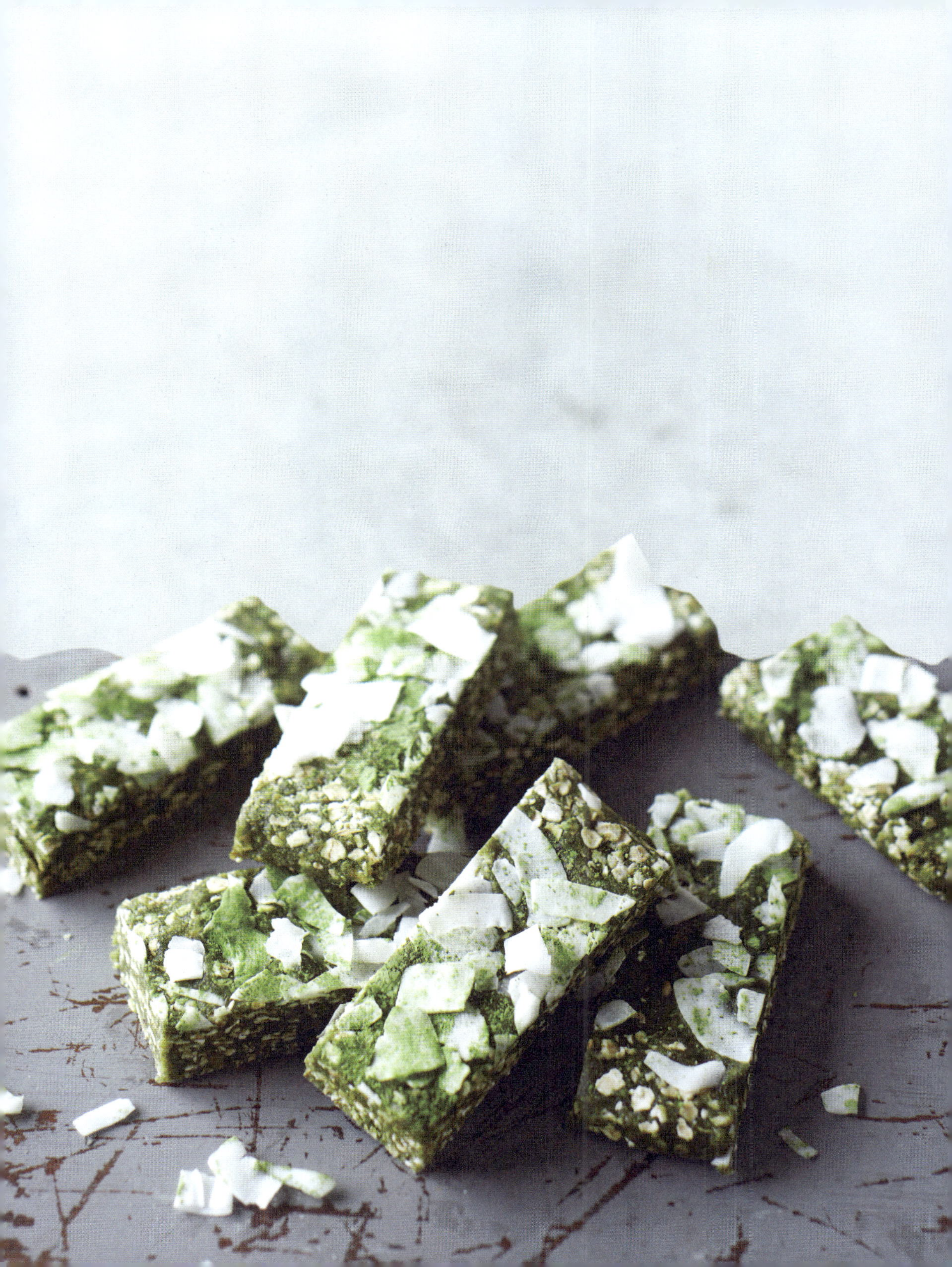

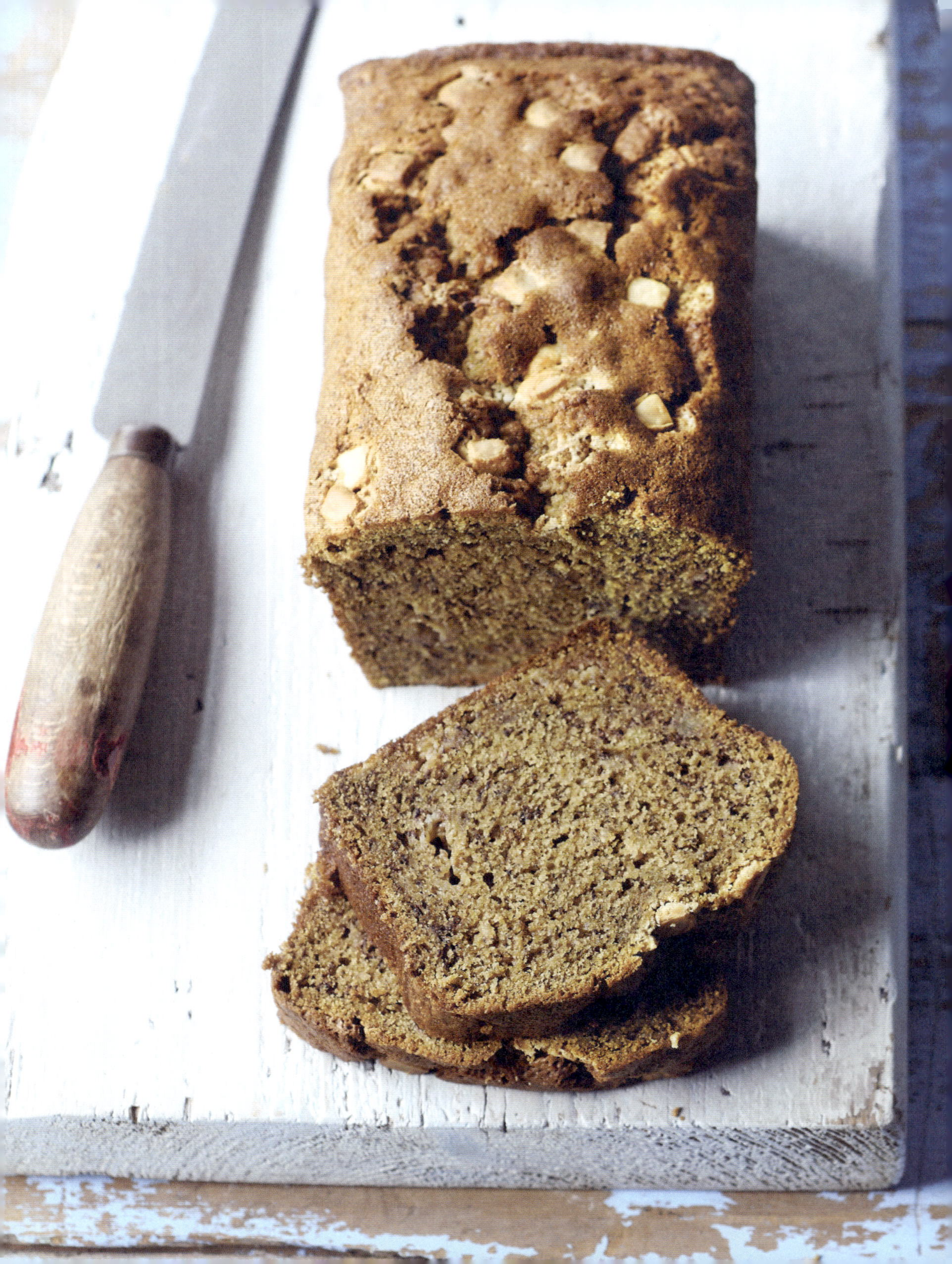

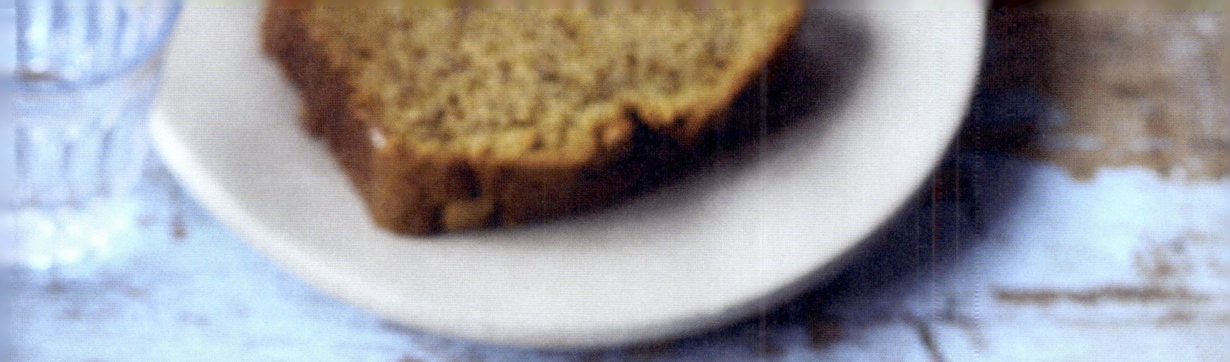

Matcha banana bread

Packed with slow-releasing energy and potassium from the bananas, this is so moreish and yummy we just had to share it with you . . .

200g (1 cup) plain (all-purpose) flour
1 tsp bicarbonate of (baking) soda
1 tsp matcha powder
½ tsp salt
125g (1 stick) salted butter
200g (1 cup) light brown sugar
2 eggs
3–4 ripe bananas
2 tbsp milk
2 tbsp natural yoghurt
1 tsp vanilla extract
50g (2oz) white chocolate chips

1 Preheat the oven to 160°C fan/180°C/350°F/gas mark 4. Grease a 23 x 12cm (9 x 4¾ inch) loaf tin and line with baking parchment.

2 Sift the flour, bicarbonate of soda, matcha powder and salt into a bowl and set aside.

3 Melt the butter, then using a hand-held electric whisk, whisk the butter with the brown sugar in a large bowl until pale and fluffy. Add the eggs, one at a time, and beat well.

4 Mash the bananas, then add to the butter and sugar mix. Mix well, then stir in the milk, yoghurt and vanilla extract. Gently mix in the dry ingredients and lastly add the chocolate chips, mixing well.

5 Pour into the prepared loaf tin and bake in the oven for 35–45 minutes or until a skewer inserted into the centre comes out clean and the loaf springs back to the touch. Leave to cool for 10–15 minutes and then enjoy!

Matcha marshmallows

These fun marshmallows are great served with chocolate or raspberry sauce. For extra green, add a little matcha powder to the icing (confectioner's) sugar and cornflour (cornstarch) mix.

MAKES ABOUT 36 MARSHMALLOWS

450g (2 cups) granulated sugar
1 tbsp liquid glucose
350ml (1½ cups) water
2 egg whites
1 tbsp matcha powder
9 sheets leaf gelatine
few drops of vanilla extract
6 tbsp icing (confectioner's) sugar
3 tbsp cornflour (cornstarch)

1 Put the granulated sugar, glucose and 200ml (1 cup) water in a saucepan. Stir over a low-medium heat to dissolve the sugar and then bring to the boil.

2 When the temperature of the sugar syrup reaches 127°C/260°F on a sugar (candy) thermometer, remove the saucepan from the heat. Take care as it will be extremely hot.

3 In a large, clean, dry bowl, beat the egg whites until they form stiff peaks. Set aside.

4 Mix the matcha powder with 2 tablespoons of the remaining water in a bowl and stir until smooth. Soak the gelatine in the remaining water for about 10 minutes until softened.

5 Carefully stir the matcha mixture, gelatine and soaking liquid into the hot sugar syrup and transfer to a jug (pitcher).

6 Gradually pour the matcha syrup onto the egg whites in a thin stream, beating all the time until really shiny. Add the vanilla and continue whisking on high speed for 8–10 minutes until the mixture holds its shape. This is best done in a food mixer, but you can use a hand-held electric whisk.

7 Lightly oil a 20 x 20cm (8 x 8in) cake tin (pan) and line with baking parchment. Combine the icing sugar and cornflour and sift some over the baking parchment.

8 Transfer the marshmallow mixture to the cake tin. Use your wet hands or a damp (step-) palette knife to press down and level the top. Dust with a little more of the sugar mixture. Chill in the fridge for 1–2 hours until set.

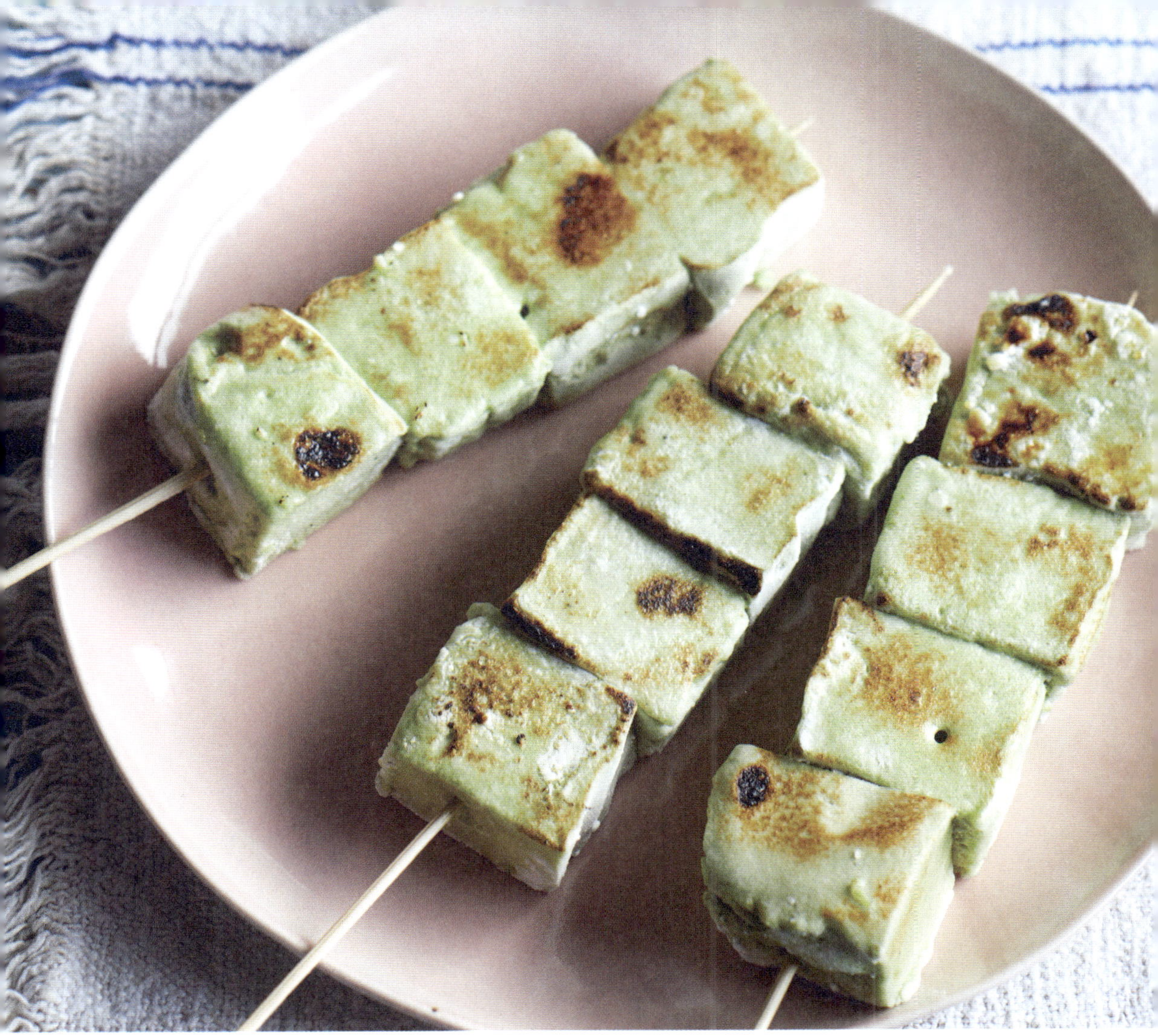

9 Carefully turn out the marshmallow onto a work surface dusted with the remaining icing sugar and cornflour. Cut into squares and roll them in the sugar mixture until thoroughly coated. Store in an airtight container in a cool, dry place.

10 To serve, thread the marshmallows onto skewers and cook under a hot grill (broiler) for 1–2 minutes until toasted.

Raw matcha coconut fudge bites

If you love chocolate, why not add some cocoa powder to the mix, or even some cacao nibs. Alternatively, dust the fudge squares with unsweetened cocoa powder.

MAKES ABOUT 20 BITE-SIZED SQUARES

6 tbsp coconut oil
175g (2 cups) unsweetened desiccated coconut, plus extra for sprinkling
4–5 tbsp agave syrup
few drops of vanilla extract
pinch of fine sea salt
2 tsp matcha powder

1 Line a small square cake tin (brownie pan) with baking parchment.

2 Melt the coconut oil in a small saucepan over a low heat.

3 Put the desiccated coconut, most of the syrup, vanilla, sea salt and matcha powder in a food processor or blender and pulse with the melted coconut oil until well mixed and there are no clumps of matcha powder. If it's not sweet enough for your taste, add some more syrup.

4 Spoon the mixture into the lined tin and press down well to level the top. Chill in the fridge for 1–2 hours until firm.

5 Cut the fudge into squares and remove from the tin. Sprinkle with desiccated coconut and store in a sealed container in the fridge, or you can freeze it.

VARIATIONS

- Substitute maple or coconut syrup for the agave syrup.
- Experiment by using coconut butter or even almond butter instead of coconut oil.

Tip

Because coconut oil melts and becomes liquid in a warm room, you must keep the fudge in the freezer or fridge.

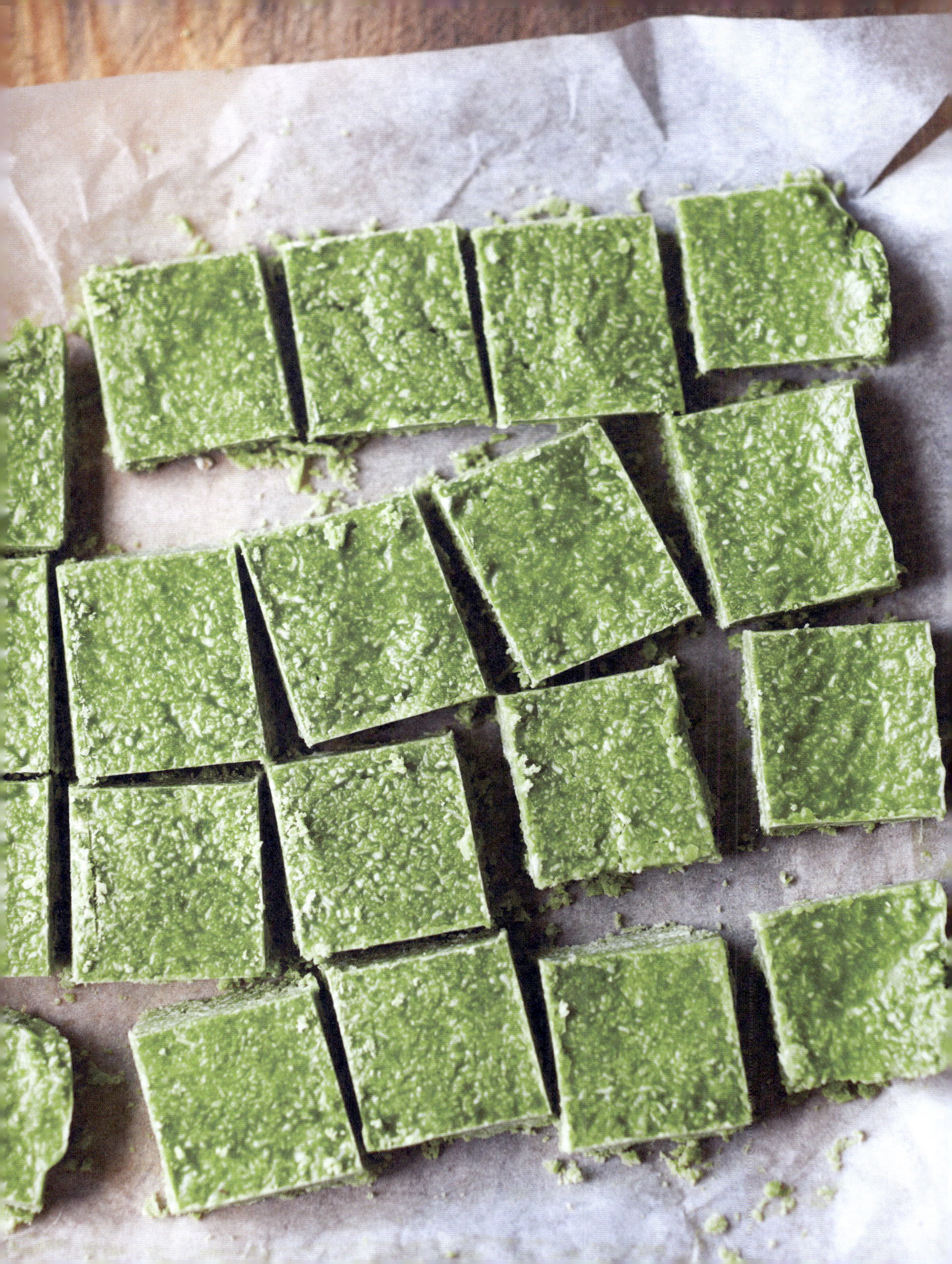

Main meals

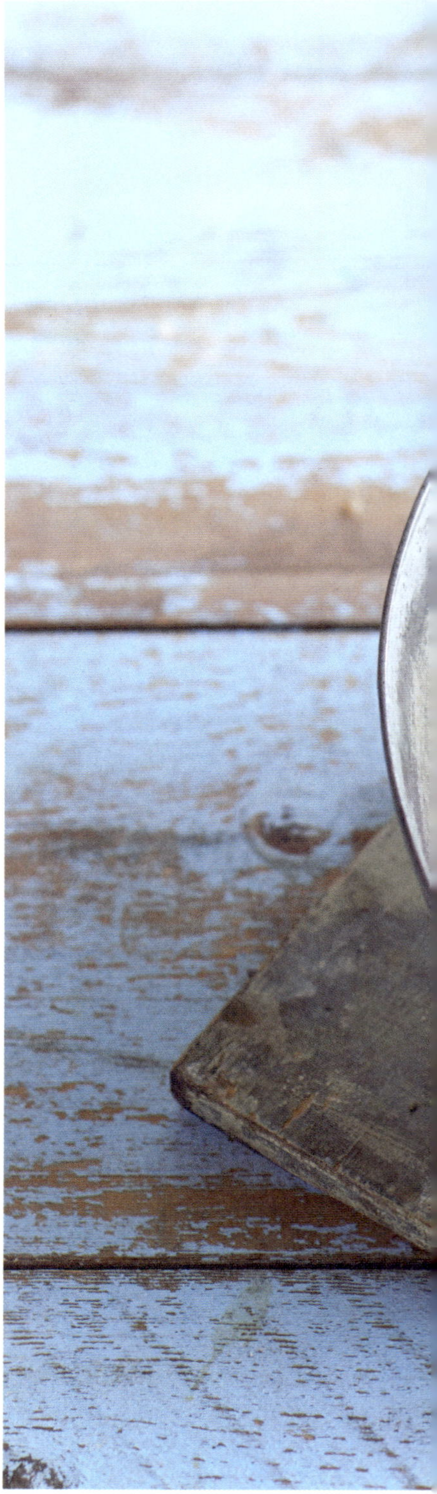

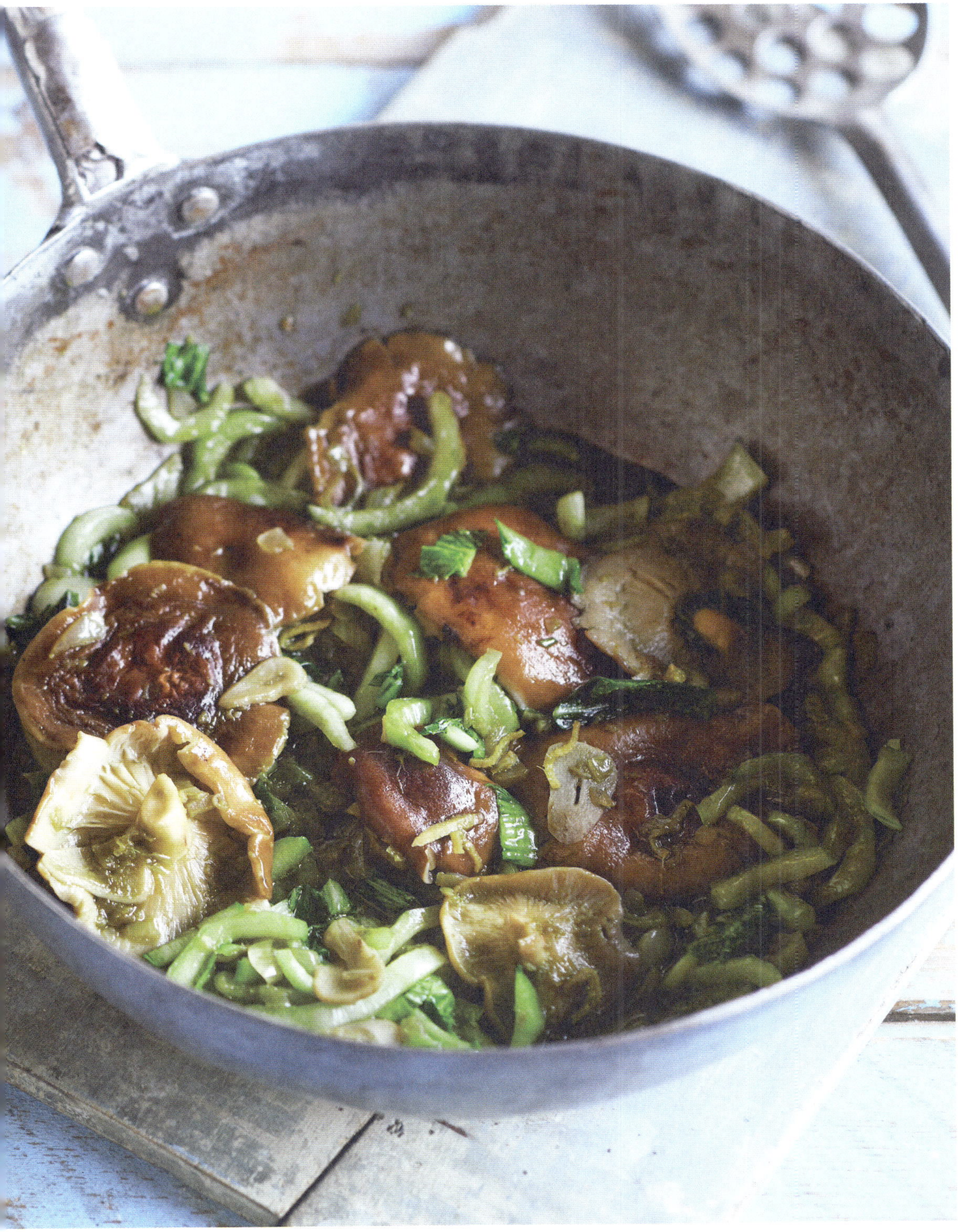

Quinoa salad with matcha chilli dressing

An extremely versatile summer salad – instead of quinoa you can use couscous or bulghur wheat, or try adding cubes of salty feta or smoked tofu.

SERVES 4

200g (1 cup) quinoa
480ml (2 cups) vegetable stock
2 tbsp olive oil
1 red onion, diced
1 large ripe avocado, peeled, stoned (pitted) and diced
60g (2oz) rocket (arugula)
handful of coriander (cilantro), chopped
small bunch of chives, snipped
salt and freshly ground black pepper
2 tbsp mixed pumpkin and sunflower seeds, to serve

FOR THE MATCHA CHILLI DRESSING

juice of 1 lemon
½ tsp matcha powder
1 small red chilli, deseeded and finely chopped
few drops of runny honey
4 tbsp olive oil

1 Rinse the quinoa under running cold water, then drain. Bring the stock to the boil in a saucepan and then add the quinoa. Reduce the heat, cover the saucepan and simmer gently for 15 minutes until the quinoa is tender and most of the stock has been absorbed. When the quinoa is cooked, the 'sprouts' or 'tails' will pop out of the seeds.

2 Remove from the heat and leave to steam in the pan for 6–8 minutes before draining off the excess liquid. Fluff up the quinoa with a fork.

3 Stir in the olive oil, red onion, avocado, rocket, coriander and chives. Season to taste with salt and pepper.

4 To make the dressing, mix together the lemon juice and matcha powder until thoroughly amalgamated. Stir in the chilli and honey, then whisk in the oil. Alternatively, shake everything together in a screwtop jar.

5 Toss the quinoa salad in the dressing until everything is coated. Sprinkle with the pumpkin and sunflower seeds and serve.

VARIATIONS

- Use orange juice, not lemon, in the dressing and add some grated fresh ginger or crushed garlic.
- Most soft herbs work well, such as parsley, basil or mint.
- Try adding grilled vegetables, e.g. beetroot (beets), asparagus, (bell) pepper, courgette (zucchini) and aubergine (eggplant).

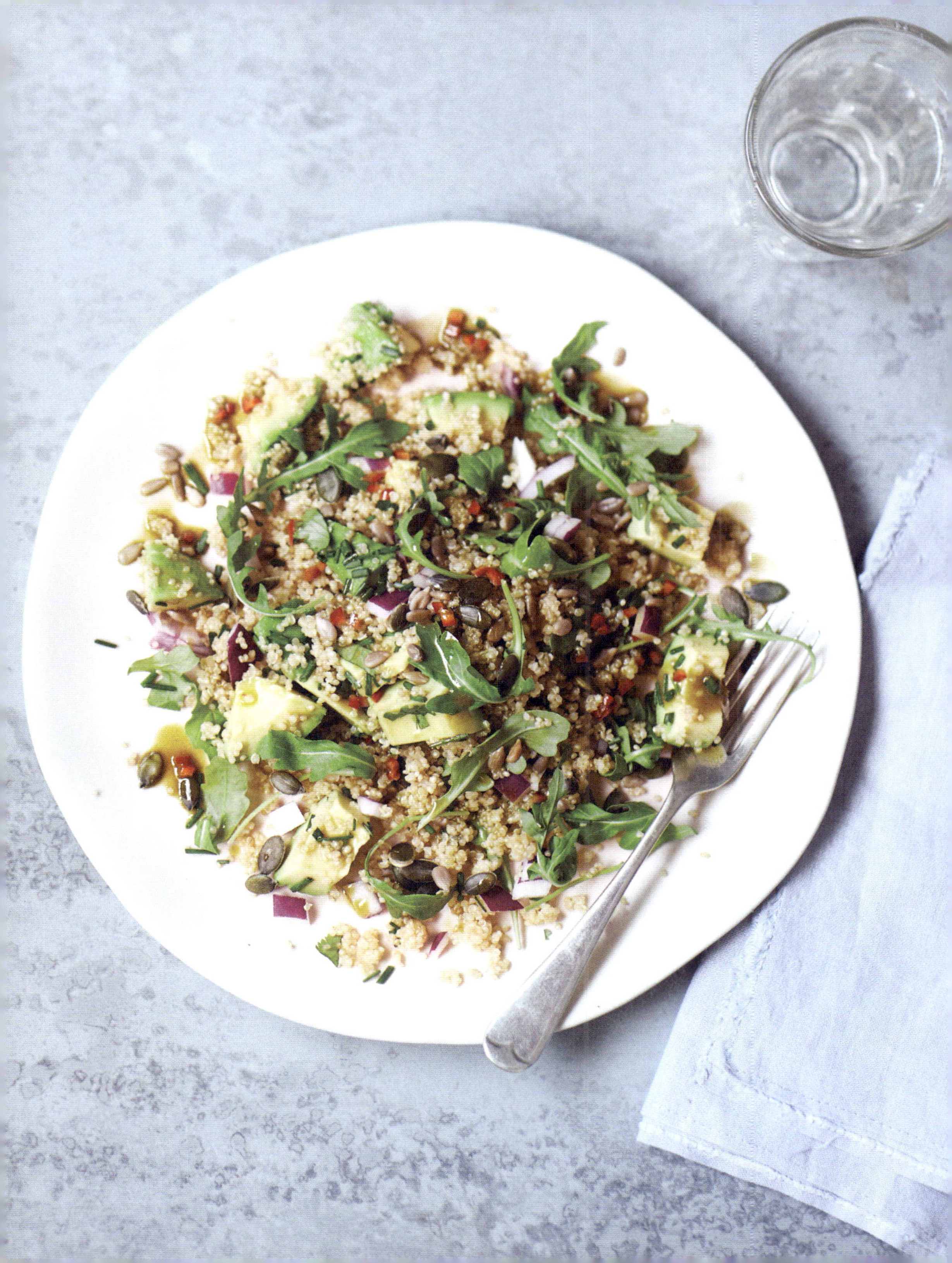

Matcha poached salmon, broccoli and chickpea salad

'This delicious salad combines salmon, which is rich in omega-3 fats, with the flavonoid-rich matcha, both of which show promise as "brain foods", with the potential to stave off cognitive decline.'

SERVES 2

FOR THE SALMON
200ml (1 cup) water, plus 1 tbsp for the paste
pinch of chilli (red pepper) flakes
½ tsp black peppercorns
½ lemon, thinly sliced
1 tsp matcha powder
50ml (¼ cup) mirin
2 salmon fillets, each about 125g (4½oz), skin on

FOR THE SALAD
8 long-stemmed broccoli
2 slices of lemon
4 handfuls of spinach leaves
1 x 400g (14oz) can chickpeas, drained and rinsed
4 spring onions (scallions), chopped

FOR THE DRESSING
4 tbsp nam pla (Thai fish sauce)
½ tsp matcha powder
juice of 2 limes
2 tbsp sweet chilli sauce
1 Thai bird's eye red chilli, deseeded and finely diced

TO SERVE
lemon wedges (optional)

1 To poach the salmon, pour the measured water into a large, deep, lidded frying pan (skillet), then add the chilli flakes and black peppercorns to the water. Bring the water to the boil over a high heat, then reduce the heat to low. Add the lemon slices.

2 Meanwhile, add the matcha to 1 tbsp of hot (not boiling) water in a small bowl or jug and whisk to make a paste.

3 Add the matcha paste to the simmering water and stir until mixed. Add the mirin, then place the salmon in the frying pan, skin-side down. Cover and leave to cook for 8 minutes, then remove from the poaching liquid and discard the liquid.

4 Meanwhile, bring some water to the boil in a steamer and steam the broccoli and lemon slices in the top of the steamer for 7 minutes, then remove from the heat.

5 To make the dressing, in a large bowl whisk half the nam pla with the matcha powder until combined. Then add the rest of the dressing ingredients and mix well.

6 To make the salad, divide the spinach, chickpeas and spring onions between two serving plates, then top with the steamed broccoli, discarding the lemon slices.

7 Top the salad with the dressing, keeping a little aside to drizzle over the salmon. Flake the salmon, discarding the skin and checking there are no bones, then place on top of the salad and drizzle over the remaining dressing. Serve with lemon wedges, if wished.

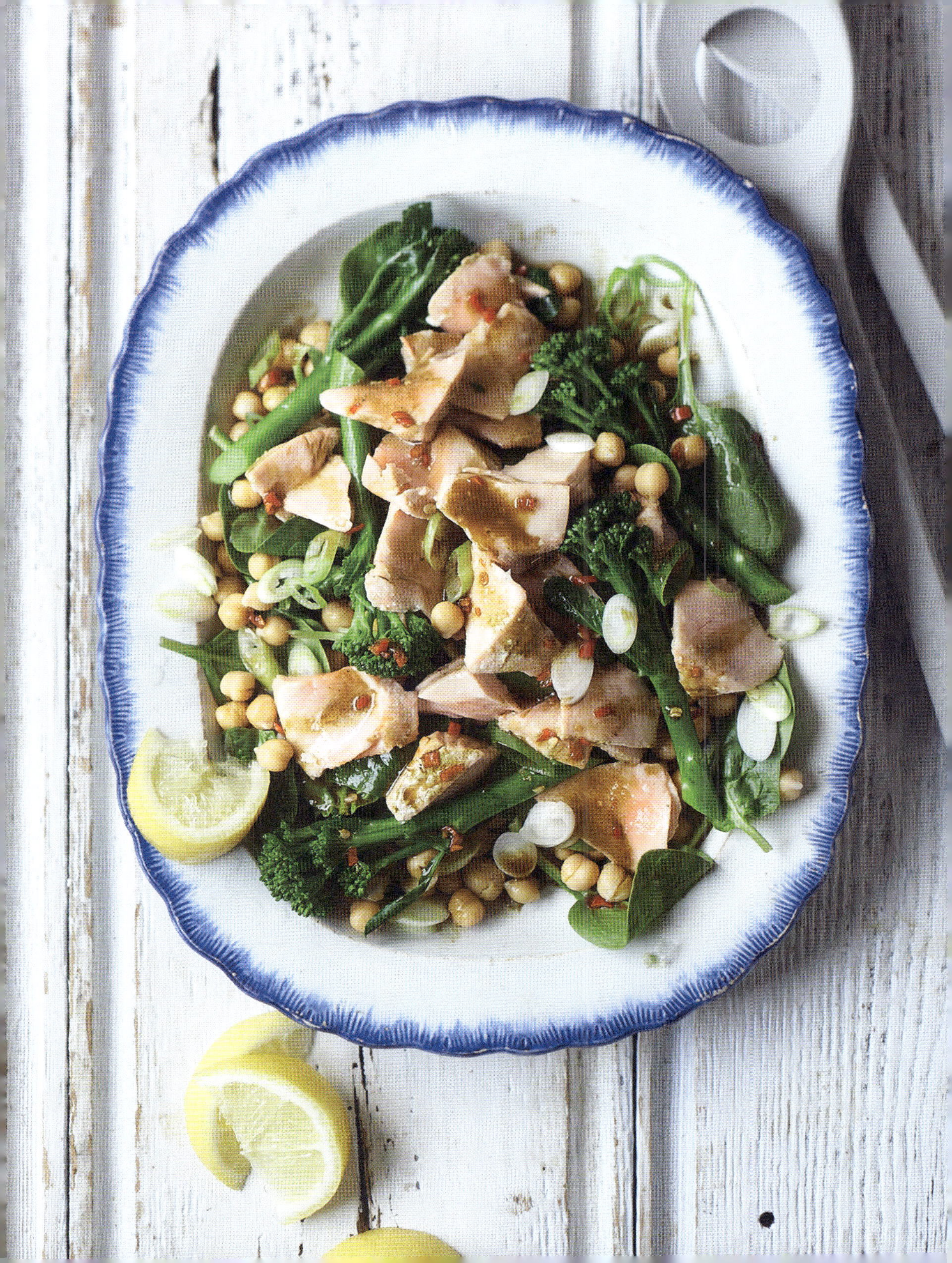

Prawn satay salad with matcha dressing

'This is a lean and mean protein-rich salad that doesn't scrimp on plant goodness. It's light, refreshing, fruity and crunchy, and the matcha satay dressing gives it a moreish creaminess.'

SERVES 4

FOR THE SATAY MARINADE, DRESSING AND PRAWNS

1 tsp matcha powder
4 tsp soy sauce
2 garlic cloves, crushed
2.5cm (1 inch) piece of fresh root ginger, peeled and grated
4 tsp smooth, all-natural peanut butter (no added salt, sugar or oil)
4 tsp hoisin sauce
juice of 1 lime
1 tsp runny honey
300g (10oz) raw prawns (shrimp)
3 tbsp coconut milk

FOR THE SALAD

2 carrots
¼ cucumber
1 apple, grated
2 celery sticks, finely sliced widthways
4 spring onions, (scallions) chopped
100g (4oz) rocket (arugula)
2 tsp sesame seeds
2 tsp pumpkin seeds

1 To make the satay marinade and dressing, add the matcha to the soy sauce in a bowl or jug (pitcher) and whisk well. Add the garlic, ginger, peanut butter, hoisin sauce, lime juice and honey, and stir really well.

2 Divide the mixture in half and use one half to marinate the prawns. Simply spread the marinade over the prawns in a large container and set aside. Reserve the other half of the mixture to make the dressing.

3 To make the salad, peel the carrots and then, using a potato peeler, peel the carrots and cucumber into long thin strips/ribbons. Mix the ribbons with the grated apple, celery and spring onions.

4 Divide the rocket between four serving plates or dishes, then top with the cucumber and apple mix. Sprinkle the sesame and pumpkin seeds over the top.

5 Finish the dressing. Simply add the coconut milk to the reserved dressing, mix well and drizzle over the salad.

6 Finally, heat a wok or deep frying pan (skillet) until hot, add the prawns along with their marinade, and stir-fry for 5 minutes. When cooked, add to the salad plates and serve straight away.

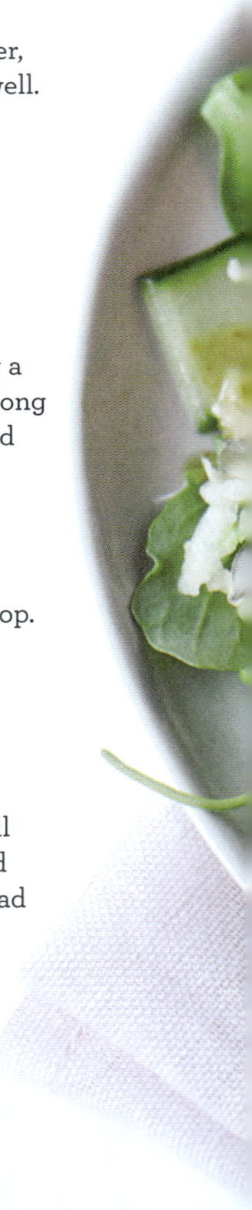

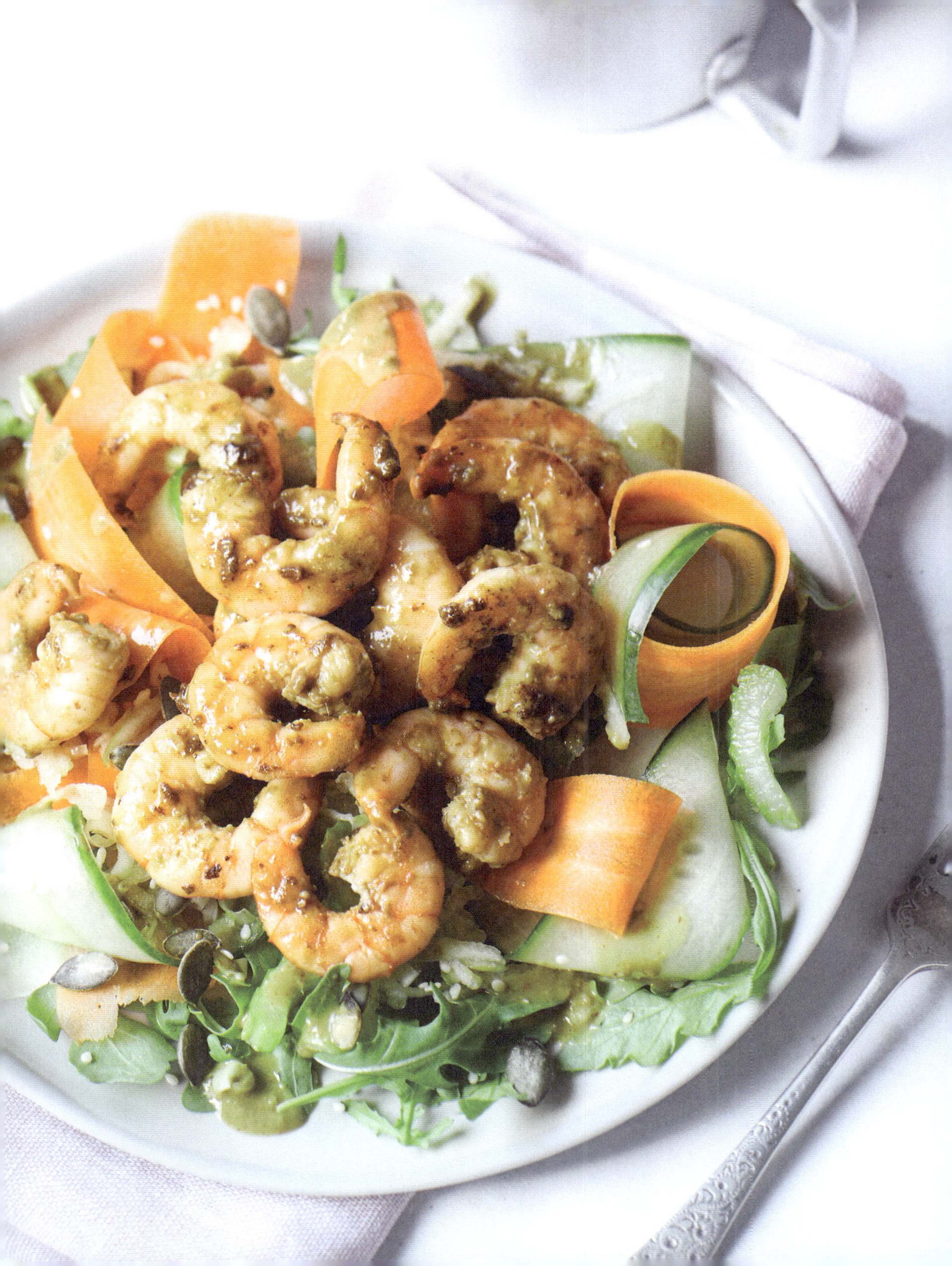

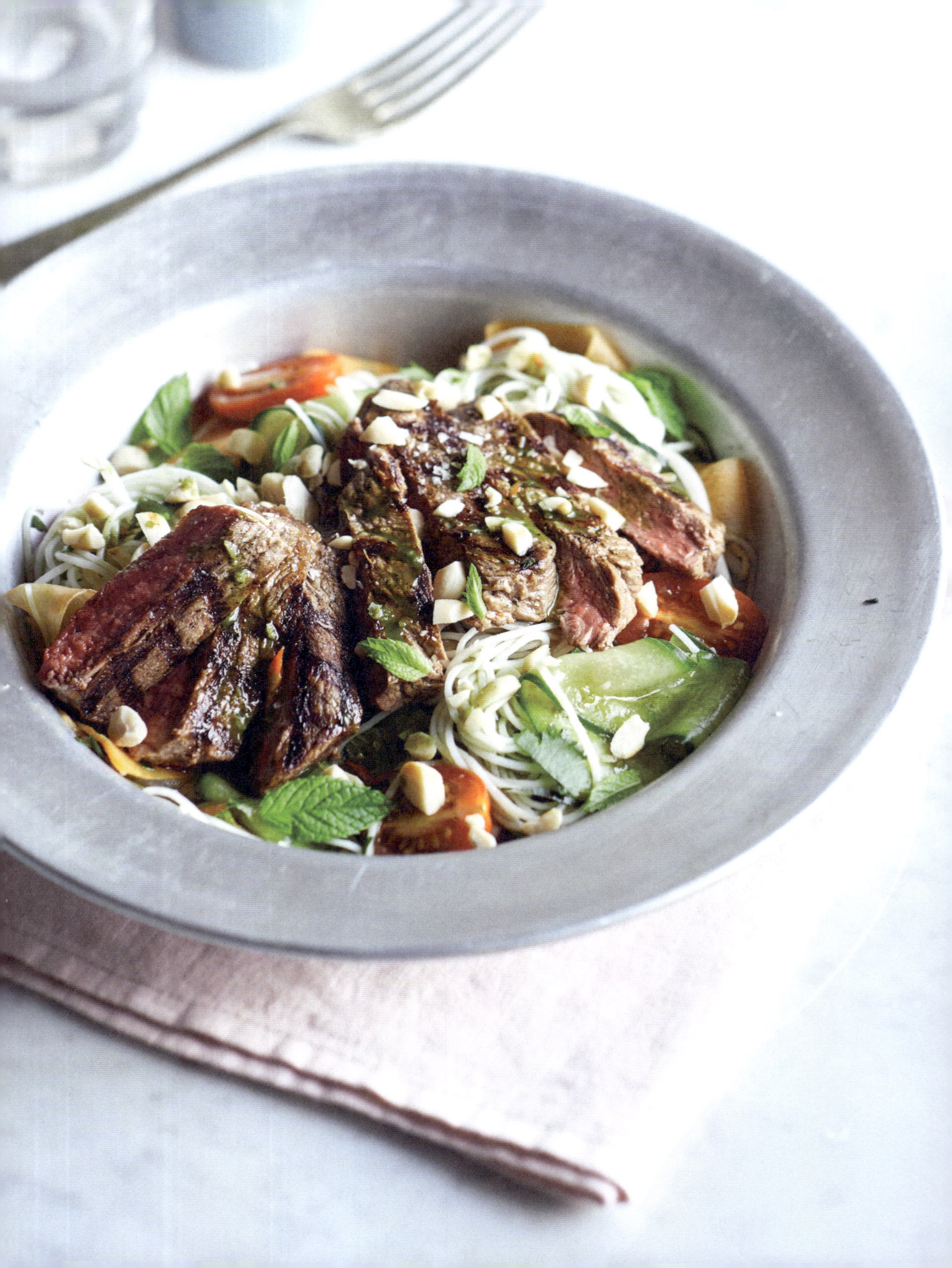

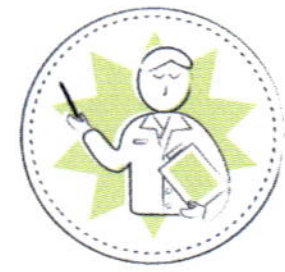

Steak and noodle salad with matcha dressing

Bursting with flavour from the fresh herbs, chillies and limes. If you don't want to use steak, this vibrant salad also works well with chicken, king prawns (jumbo shrimp) or salmon.

SERVES 4

250g (9oz) rice noodles
2 large carrots
½ cucumber
6 fresh lime leaves, stems and central veins removed
300g (10oz) bean sprouts
1 small bunch of coriander (cilantro), roughly chopped
handful of mint, chopped
8 cherry tomatoes, halved
3 lean sirloin (strip loin) steaks, visible fat removed
pinch of sea salt
6 tbsp unsalted peanuts, toasted and chopped

FOR THE MATCHA DRESSING
juice of 1 lime
2 tbsp nam pla (Thai fish sauce)
1 tsp light soy sauce
1 garlic clove, crushed
pinch of caster (superfine) sugar
1 red Thai bird's eye chilli, deseeded and shredded
1 tsp matcha powder

1 Put the rice noodles in a bowl and cover with cold water. Leave them to soak for about 15 minutes, until softened. Drain well and set aside.

2 Peel the carrots and then, using a potato peeler, peel them into long thin strips. Cut the cucumber in half and discard the seeds. Use a potato peeler to cut it into long strips. Roll up the lime leaves and shred them as thinly as possible.

3 Put the carrots, cucumber, lime leaves, bean sprouts, coriander, mint and tomatoes in a serving dish.

4 Mix all the dressing ingredients together, whisking in the matcha powder a little at a time until well combined and no clumps remain. Alternatively, shake everything vigorously in a screwtop jar.

5 Cook the steaks on a lightly oiled hot griddle or ridged grill pan until appetizingly charred on the outside but still pink inside. Slice them thickly and sprinkle with sea salt.

6 Add the rice noodles to the vegetables and toss gently in the dressing. Divide between four plates and add the strips of steak. Sprinkle with the peanuts and serve immediately while the steak is still warm.

VARIATIONS

- Try adding a spoonful of sweet chilli sauce to the dressing or drizzle some over the top.
- Rocket (arugula) or watercress are healthy additions and add a peppery flavour. Or try baby spinach leaves or finely shredded kale.

Matcha gnocchi with sage and orange sauce

Perfect for a chilly autumn night, try adding a pinch of grated nutmeg to the flour and matcha when making the gnocchi for a more distinctive, subtly spicy flavour.

SERVES 4

500g (1lb 2oz) Désirée (Yukon Gold) potatoes, washed and dried
175g (1½ cups) plain (all-purpose) flour, plus extra for dusting
pinch of salt
1 tbsp matcha powder
1 egg, beaten
grated Parmesan, to serve
snipped chives, to serve

FOR THE SAGE AND ORANGE SAUCE

100g (½ cup) butter
6 sage leaves
juice of 1 large orange
salt and freshly ground black pepper

1 Preheat the oven to 170°C fan/190°C/375°F/gas mark 5.

2 To make the gnocchi, prick the potatoes all over with a skewer and place on a baking tray (sheet). Cook in the preheated oven for about 1 hour, until tender. Remove from the oven and leave to cool.

3 When the potatoes are cool enough to handle, remove the skins.

4 On a clean work surface, sprinkle about two-thirds of the flour plus the salt and matcha powder. Push the potatoes through a fine sieve or a potato ricer and add to the flour. Make a well in the centre and add the beaten egg. Mix everything together with your hands, gradually adding more flour as and when needed. You should end up with a soft dough. Do not over-mix.

5 Roll out or flatten the dough to a square, about 1.5cm (½in) thick, on a clean, floured work surface. Cut it into 1.5cm (½in) wide strips and roll each one into a long cylindrical sausage shape. Next, cut each sausage into smaller pieces, dust lightly with flour and then press each one lightly with the tines of a fork to leave indentations.

6 To make the sauce, melt the butter over a low heat in a large frying pan (skillet). Add the sage leaves and heat through for 1 minute, allowing the flavour to infuse the sauce. Stir in the orange juice and season to taste with salt and pepper. Remove and discard the sage leaves.

7 Bring a large saucepan of water to the boil, then reduce the heat to a bare simmer. Add the gnocchi and give them a gentle stir. When they all rise to the surface and float, count to 10 and then remove with a slotted spoon.

8 Add the gnocchi to the hot sauce and divide between four serving plates. Sprinkle with Parmesan and chives and serve immediately.

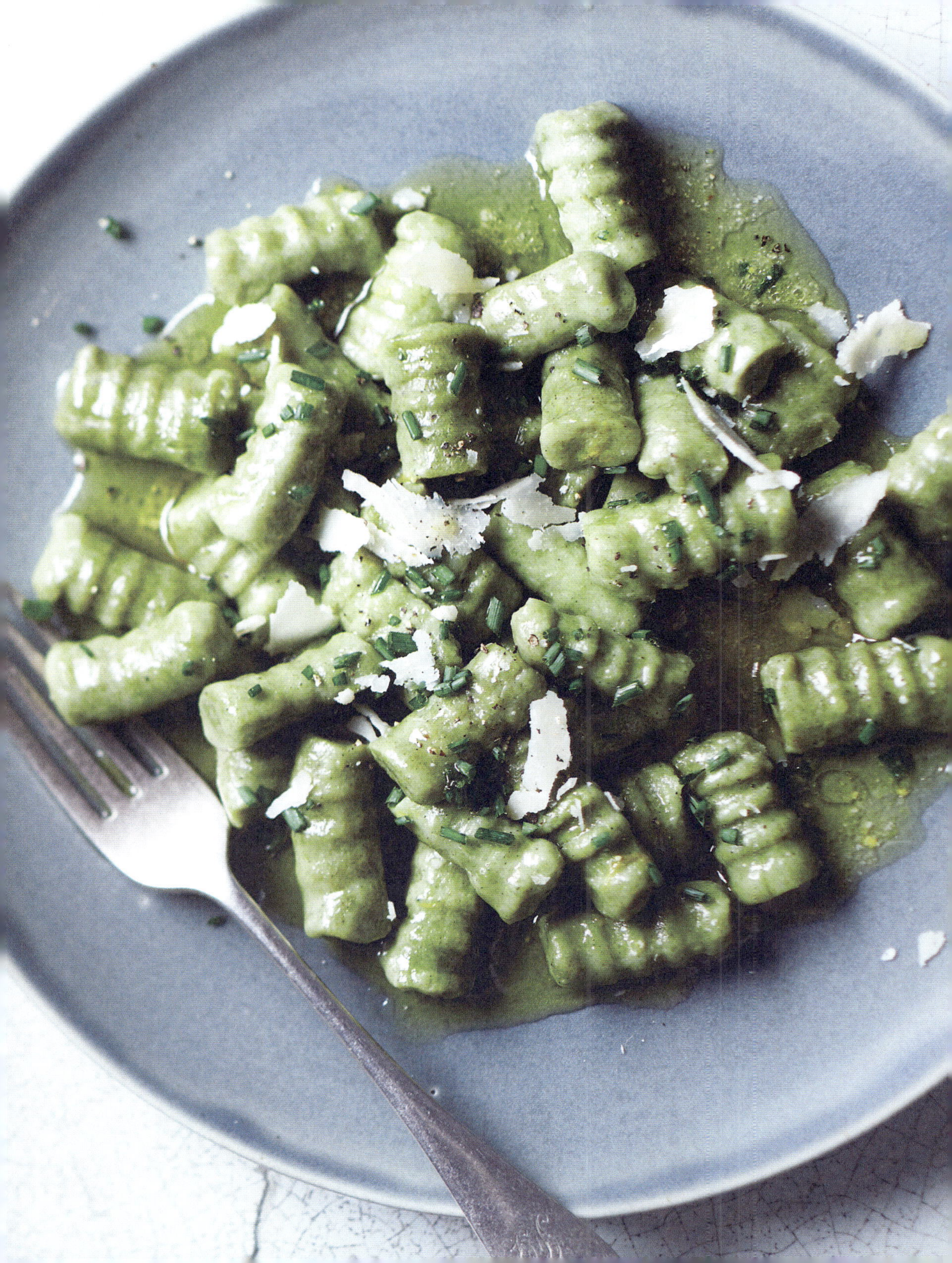

Shiitake, pak choi and matcha teriyaki stir-fry

Here we've included another treasured Japanese food in a dish that indulges your immune system. 'Shiitake is classified as a "medicinal mushroom" and extensively studied for its potent immune – and wellness – enhancing effects.'

SERVES 2

FOR THE TERIYAKI SAUCE

1 tbsp runny honey
2 tbsp light soy sauce
2 tbsp water
2 tbsp sesame oil
2 tbsp fresh root ginger, peeled and grated
1 garlic clove, chopped
1 tsp matcha powder

FOR THE STIR-FRY

1 tbsp coconut oil
4cm (1½ inch) piece of fresh root ginger, peeled and finely chopped
2 garlic cloves, finely sliced
½ onion, finely chopped
2 spring onions (scallions), finely chopped
125g (4½oz) shiitake mushrooms
3 pak choi (bok choy), chopped
steamed brown rice, to serve

1 Make the teriyaki sauce by combining all the ingredients for the sauce, stirring well so there are no lumps of matcha powder.

2 Place a large wok or deep frying pan (skillet) over a medium-high heat. Add the coconut oil, and when the pan is hot, stir-fry the ginger and garlic until soft, about 3 minutes. Add the onion and stir-fry for 2–3 minutes, then add the spring onions and cook for another minute.

3 Add the mushrooms and cook for 1 minute, then add the teriyaki sauce and stir-fry for about 5 minutes.

4 Finally add the pak choi and toss in the hot wok for about 2 minutes, then remove from the heat and serve with steamed brown rice.

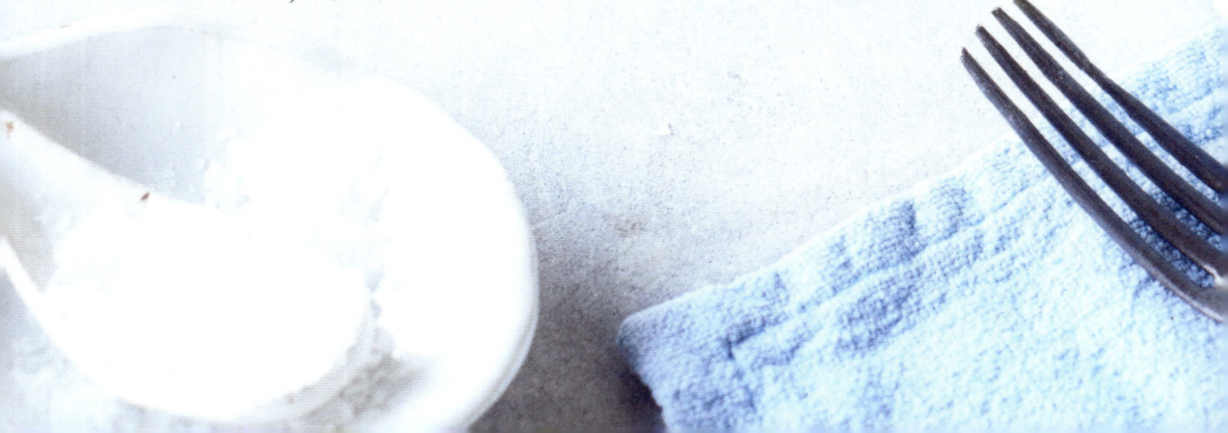

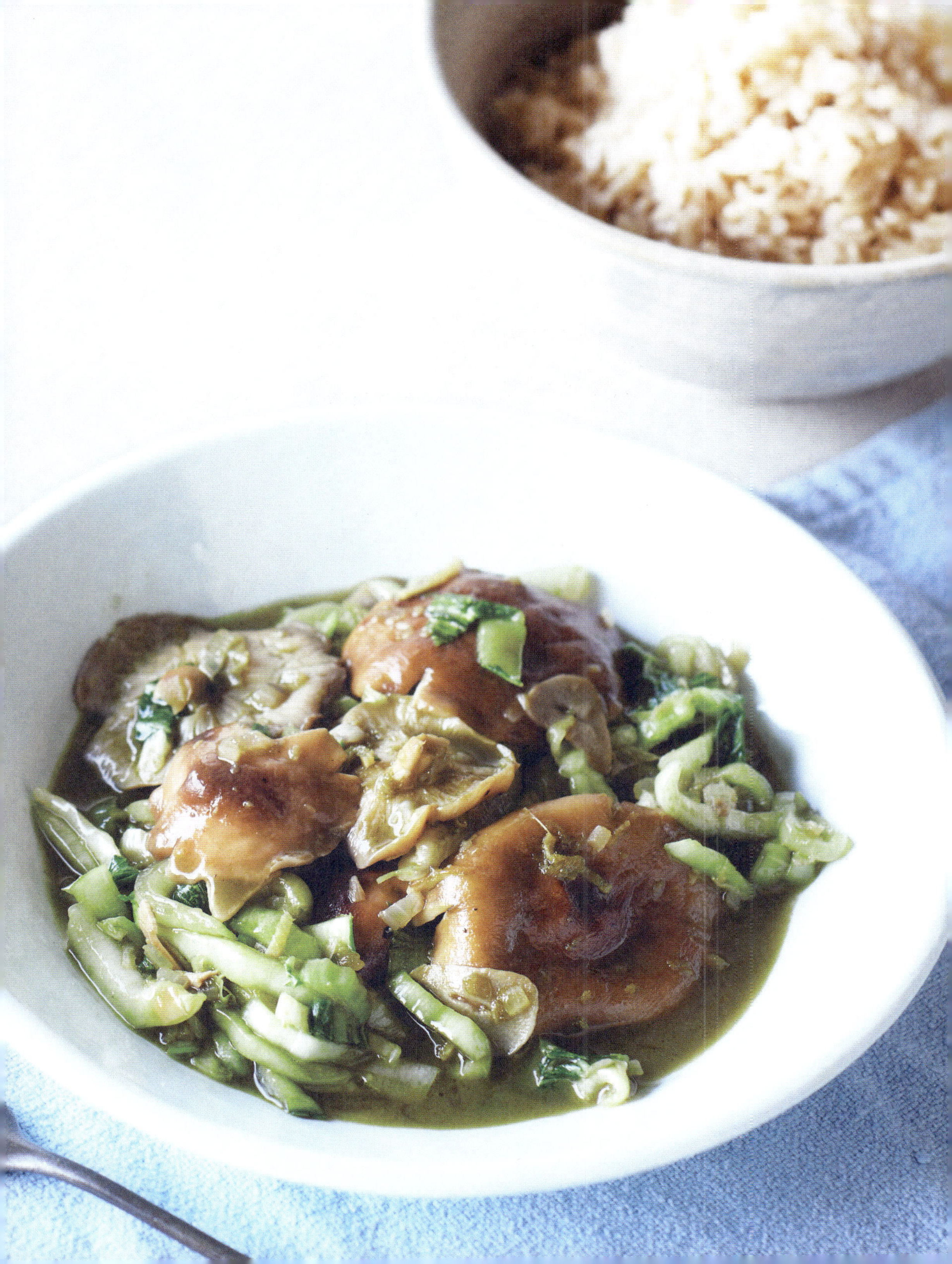

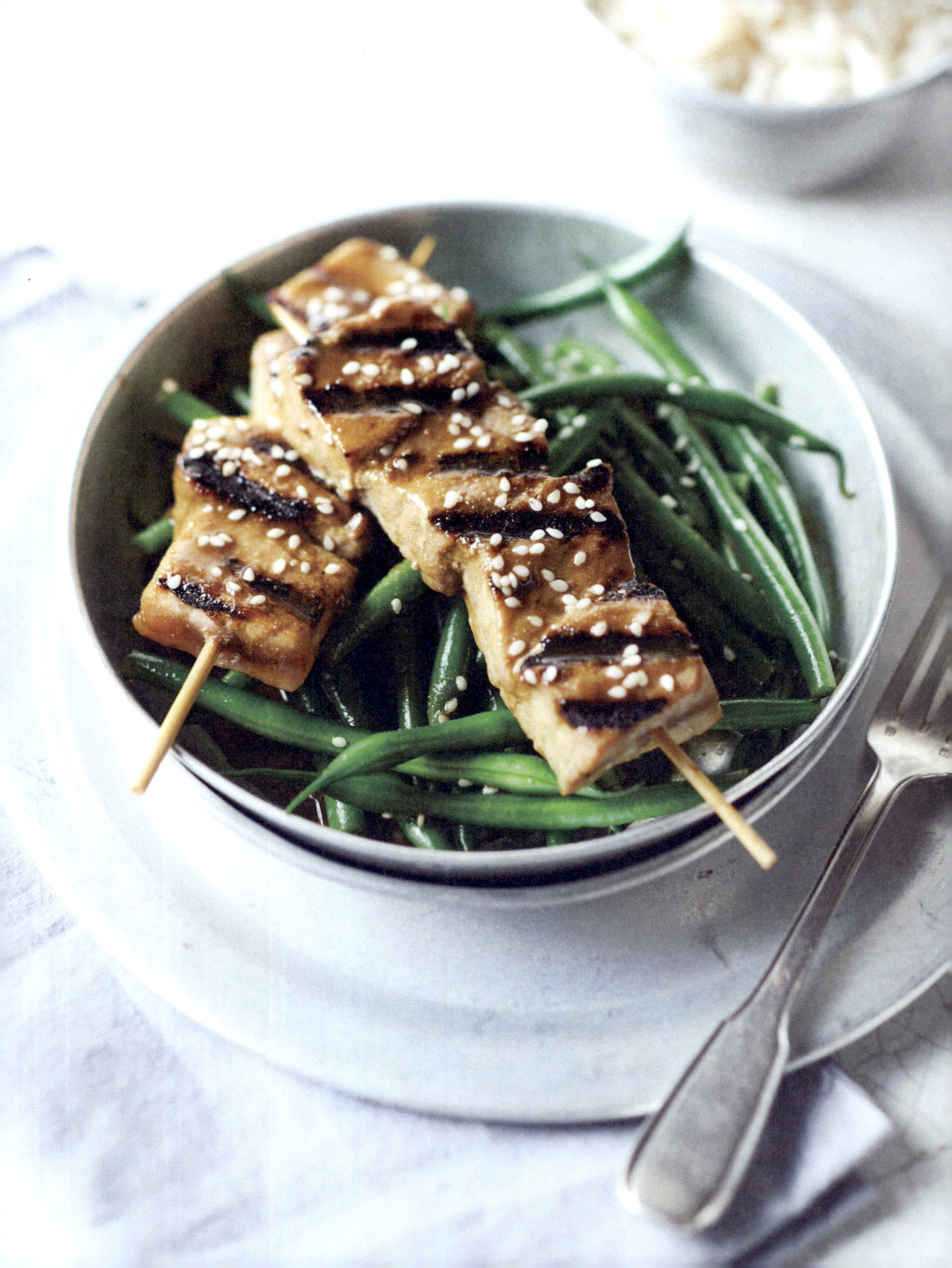

Wasabi tuna with matcha green beans

Packed with taste, this Japanese-influenced dish works equally well with fresh salmon instead of tuna, and goes well with either rice noodles or rice.

SERVES 4

400g (14oz) tuna fillet
2 tbsp soy sauce
1 tsp fresh root ginger, peeled and grated
2 tsp wasabi paste
1 tsp sesame oil, plus extra for brushing
250g (9oz) thin green beans, trimmed
sesame seeds, to serve
boiled or steamed rice, to serve

FOR THE MATCHA DRESSING

1 tbsp rice wine vinegar
1 tsp matcha powder
3 tbsp sesame oil
1 tbsp teriyaki sauce

Tip

Soaking the wooden or bamboo skewers in warm water for at least 20 minutes before use will prevent them from burning.

1 Cut the tuna into 2.5cm (1in) chunks and place in a bowl with 1 tbsp of the soy sauce. Turn the tuna pieces gently until they are coated with the sauce and then thread onto 4 wooden skewers that have been soaked in warm water (see the tip below).

2 Mix the remaining soy sauce with the ginger, wasabi paste and sesame oil.

3 To make the matcha dressing, put the vinegar in a small bowl and whisk in the matcha powder until thoroughly mixed. Whisk in the sesame oil and teriyaki sauce.

4 Steam the green beans until they are just tender but still retain some 'bite', or cook in a saucepan of boiling water. Drain well and toss immediately in the matcha dressing.

5 Heat a griddle pan over a medium-high heat and brush with a little oil. Place the tuna skewers on the hot griddle and cook for 2 minutes each side until seared all over. Sprinkle with the wasabi mixture and cook for 1 minute. The tuna should be slightly pink on the inside and seared outside. If you like it more well done, cook for another minute.

6 Serve the tuna skewers, sprinkled with sesame seeds, on a bed of the matcha green beans with rice to accompany.

VARIATIONS

- Cook the tuna steaks on the griddle instead of making them into kebabs, but note that they will take longer to cook as steaks.
- Vary the green vegetables – why not try steamed pak choi (bok choy) or Chinese cabbage.

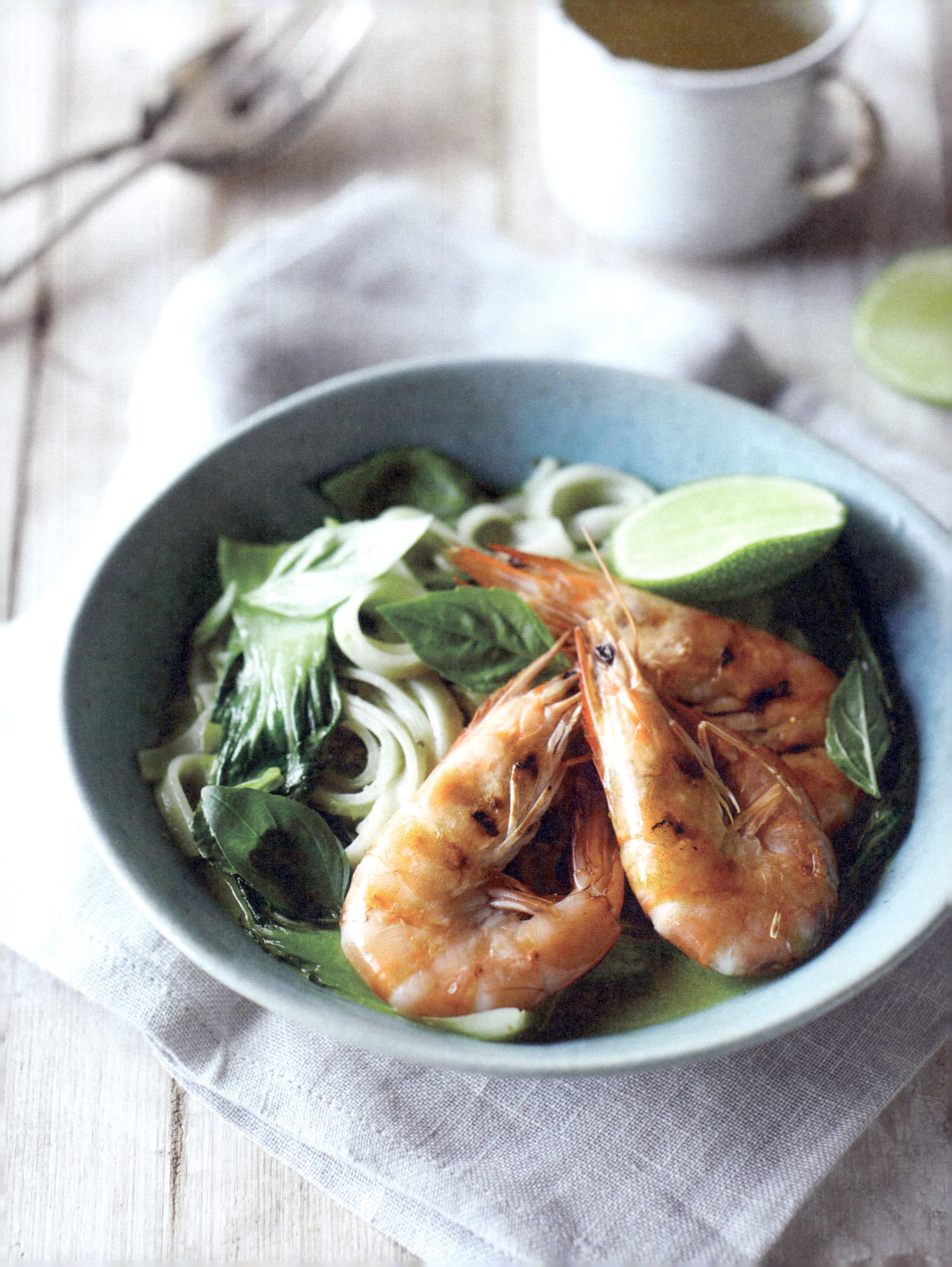

Matcha Thai green curry with king prawns

This is a take on the classic Thai green curry – it is delightfully creamy and coconutty with a subtle taste of matcha green tea.

SERVES 4

400g (14oz) rice noodles
oil, for grilling
1 tbsp coconut oil
2 garlic cloves, crushed
5cm (2in) piece of fresh root ginger, peeled and diced
1 lemongrass stalk, peeled and thinly sliced
1 bunch spring onions (scallions), thinly sliced
450g (1lb) baby pak choi (bok choy), shredded
2 tsp matcha powder
300ml (1¼ cups) chicken stock, warmed
600ml (2½ cups) reduced-fat coconut milk
grated zest and juice of 1 lime
2 tsp nam pla (Thai fish sauce)
1 tbsp Thai green curry paste
1 tbsp coconut palm sugar
500g (17½oz) raw king prawns (jumbo shrimp), shell on
large handful of Thai basil, chopped
salt and freshly ground black pepper
lime wedges, to serve

1 Cook the rice noodles according to the instructions on the packet. Preheat a lightly oiled griddle pan until hot.

2 Heat the coconut oil in a large saucepan over a medium heat. Add the garlic, ginger, lemongrass, spring onions and pak choi, and cook, stirring once or twice, for 3 minutes.

3 Mix the matcha powder with a little of the warm stock, stirring well, and then add to the vegetables in the saucepan with the remaining stock and the coconut milk.

4 Add the lime zest and juice, nam pla, Thai green curry paste and palm sugar and heat through gently until piping hot.

5 Meanwhile, cook the prawns on the hot griddle pan for about 2 minutes on each side, leaving the shells on the prawns, or at least on the tails. The prawns should turn pink and be juicy. Do not overcook them or they will become tough.

6 Stir the chopped Thai basil and drained rice noodles into the curry. Season to taste with salt and pepper.

7 Ladle the curry into four shallow bowls and arrange the grilled prawns on top. Garnish with lime wedges and serve immediately.

VARIATIONS

- You can add a little heat to the broth by cooking a diced chilli with the garlic and ginger mixture in step 2 above. Or sprinkle the curry with some sliced chilli as a garnish.
- Instead of prawns, top the dish with some grilled chicken.

Chicken, turmeric, matcha and pepper casserole

'This spicy number contains powerful natural anti-inflammatory plant compounds, most notably from the turmeric. But it's the synergy of the ingredients that really amplifies these benefits. The EGCG from the matcha enhances turmeric's effects in the body, while the piperine from the black pepper, and the presence of fats, increases turmeric's absorption.'

SERVES 4

1 chicken stock cube
500g (2½ cups) puy or green lentils
500g (1lb 2oz) skinless chicken thighs, or a mixture of thighs and legs
salt
2 tbsp freshly ground black pepper
1 tbsp coconut oil
1 onion, finely chopped
2.5cm (1 inch) piece of fresh root ginger, peeled and finely chopped
2 garlic cloves, crushed
juice of ½ lemon
2 tsp ground turmeric
2 tsp matcha powder
240ml (1 cup) water, plus 2 tbsp warm water
250g (9oz) spinach leaves
flatbread, to serve

1 First prepare the lentils. Bring a saucepan of water to the boil and add the stock cube. Add the lentils and leave to cook for 20 minutes. Drain and set aside.

2 Place the chicken pieces in a large bowl and season well with salt. Then add lots of black pepper so it completely coats the chicken.

3 Over a medium heat, in a large lidded casserole dish, heat the coconut oil and then gently fry the onion, ginger and garlic. Season with a little salt and pepper.

4 Once the onion, ginger and garlic are soft, add the peppered chicken to the casserole dish and fry for 3–4 minutes until browned. The pepper should give the chicken a good, firm coating. Add the lemon juice, then the turmeric, and mix well.

5 Next add the matcha to a medium-sized bowl, add 2 tbsp of warm water and whisk well. Add the rest of the measured water to the matcha and then add the matcha to the casserole dish. Cover the casserole dish and cook over a low heat for 25 minutes, stirring occasionally so it does not stick.

6 Add the spinach and cooked lentils to the chicken curry, stir in well, and cook for 3 more minutes. Serve with flatbread.

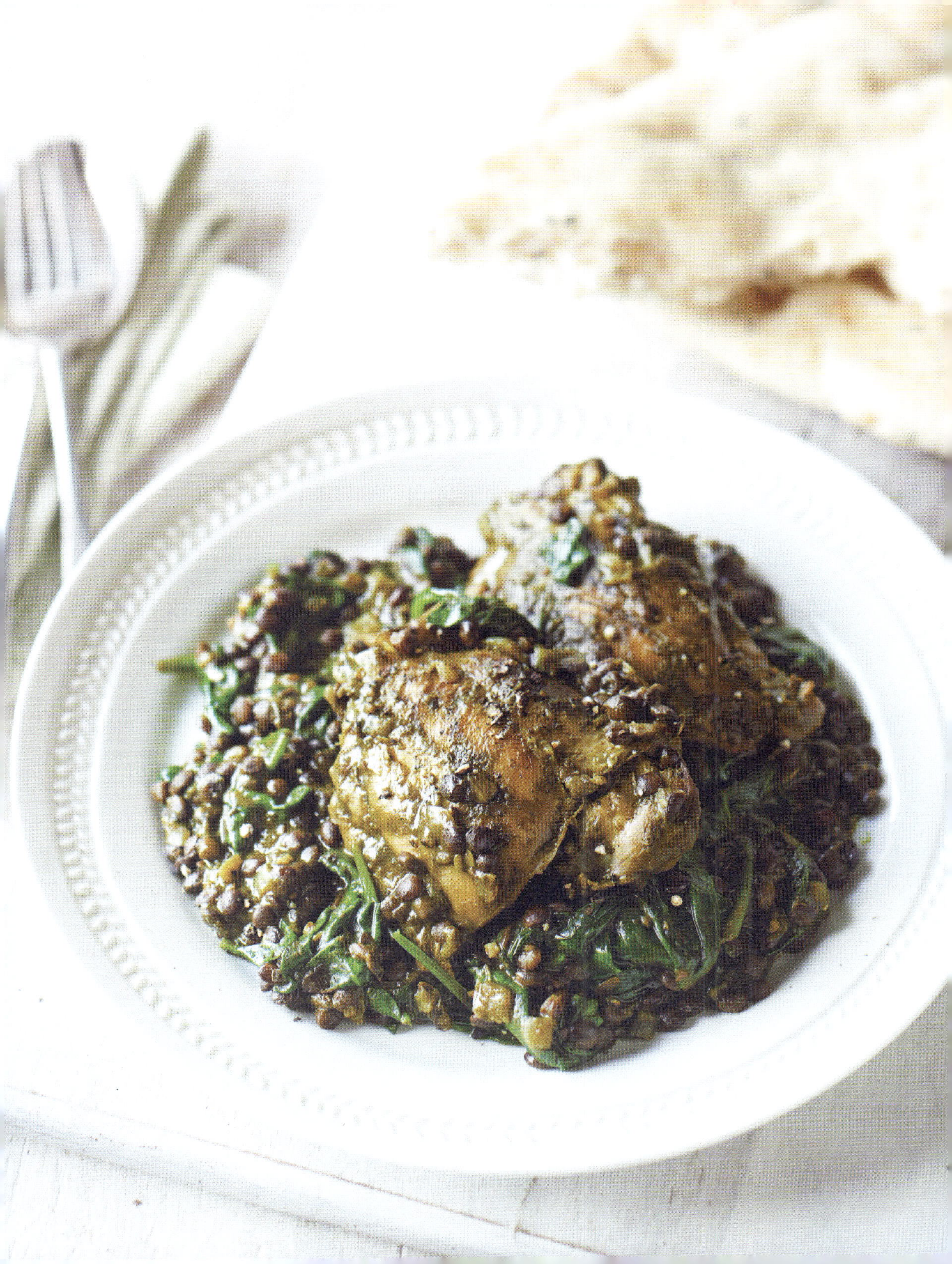

Mexican chicken with matcha guacamole

This is a great midweek dinner to share with friends, especially in the knowledge that Aidan and Glen encourage eating hot, spicy food regularly, thanks to the health benefits bestowed by chillies.

SERVES 4

grated zest and juice of 2 limes
1 tsp red chilli, deseeded and diced
2 garlic cloves, crushed
1 tbsp olive or peanut oil
4 chicken breasts, skinned and boned
1 bunch spring onions (scallions), trimmed
salt and freshly ground black pepper
tortillas, warmed, to serve

FOR THE MATCHA GUACAMOLE
1 green chilli, deseeded and diced
½ red onion, diced
1 garlic clove, crushed
¼ tsp sea salt
2 avocados
juice of 1 lime
1 small bunch of coriander (cilantro), chopped
1 tsp matcha powder
1 tomato, deseeded and diced
freshly ground black pepper

1 In a bowl, mix together the lime zest and juice, chilli, garlic and oil for the marinade. Add a grinding of salt and pepper.

2 Slash each chicken breast 3 or 4 times with a sharp knife and add to the marinade, turning until the chicken is completely coated. Set aside while you make the guacamole.

3 Crush the chilli, red onion, garlic and salt in a pestle and mortar. Cut the avocados in half and remove the stones. Scoop out the flesh and mash roughly with a fork – it shouldn't be too smooth. Stir in the lime juice. Add the coriander, crushed red onion mixture, matcha powder and tomato. Mix everything together and add a grinding of black pepper.

4 Cook the chicken on an oiled griddle pan or under a preheated hot grill (broiler) for 8–10 minutes on each side until sticky and golden brown on the outside and cooked right through inside. Remove and keep warm.

5 Add the spring onions to the hot griddle and cook for 1–2 minutes on each side until slightly charred and just tender.

6 Cut the hot chicken into slices and serve immediately with the spring onions, matcha guacamole and warmed tortillas.

VARIATIONS

- Divide the chicken between the tortillas and add some guacamole, a spoonful of hot salsa, some Greek yoghurt and griddled (bell) peppers. Roll up and eat with your hands.
- Instead of spring onions, cook some sliced red, green and yellow (bell) peppers and red onions on the griddle to serve with the chicken.

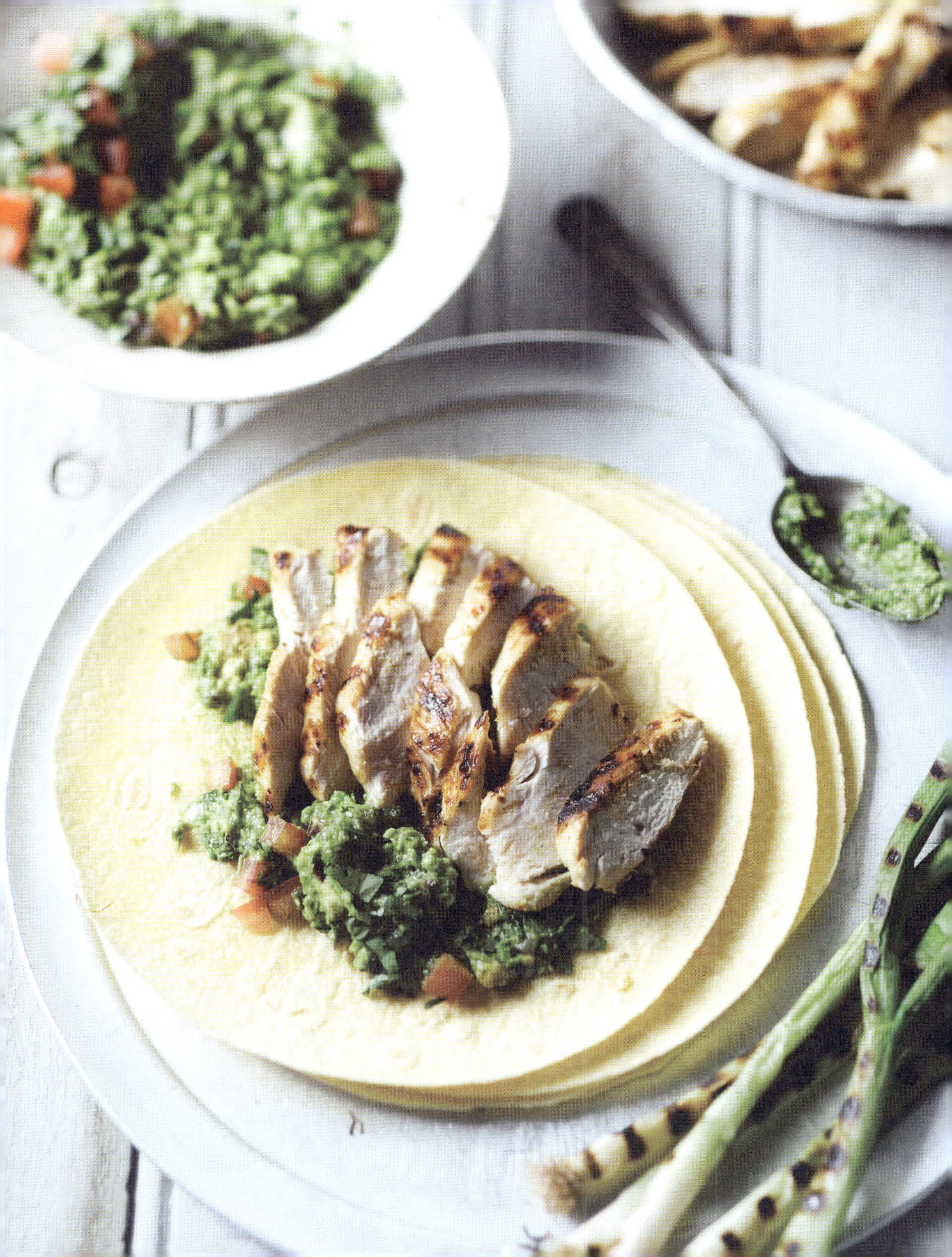

Stir-fried pork and matcha soba noodles

Our nutritionists are fans of soba noodles, which are made from buckwheat, a high-protein, nutritious and versatile gluten-free 'pseudo-grain'. Full of minerals and fibre, and great tasting, they'll soon become a storecupboard staple. For a more zingy flavour, include some grated lime zest and juice; or for a bit of crunch add cashew nuts.

SERVES 4

300g (10oz) matcha soba noodles
1 tbsp sesame oil
3 tbsp coconut oil
1 tbsp fresh root ginger, peeled and grated
1 red chilli, deseeded and diced
1 garlic clove, crushed
1 bunch spring onions (scallions), sliced diagonally
1 red (bell) pepper, deseeded and thinly sliced
300g (10oz) pak choi (bok choy), shredded
2 tbsp light soy sauce
2 tsp nam pla (Thai fish sauce)
4 tbsp chicken or vegetable stock
1 tsp caster (superfine) sugar
350g (12oz) lean pork fillet (tenderloin), thinly sliced
salt
freshly ground peppercorns (black or Szechuan)
roughly chopped coriander (cilantro), to garnish

1 Cook the noodles in a saucepan of salted boiling water according to the packet instructions. They should be just tender with a little 'bite'. Drain well.

2 Meanwhile, place a large wok or deep frying pan (skillet) over a medium-high heat. Add the sesame oil and 2 tbsp of the coconut oil. When the pan is really hot, stir-fry the ginger, chilli and garlic for 1 minute without colouring.

3 Add the spring onions, red pepper and pak choi and toss in the hot wok until the pak choi starts to wilt.

4 Stir in the drained noodles, soy sauce, nam pla, stock and sugar. Stir-fry for 2 minutes.

5 Fry the pork briskly in the remaining coconut oil in a separate frying pan over a high heat for 4–5 minutes, until golden brown on both sides and thoroughly cooked. Grind plenty of pepper over the top.

6 Divide the stir-fried noodle mixture between four serving plates and top with the pork. Sprinkle with coriander and serve immediately.

Note

If you fancy making your own matcha noodles you can follow a basic recipe for fresh egg pasta, adding 1 tbsp matcha powder per 300g (2½ cups) Tipo 00 flour. To make it easier, make the pasta in a food processor and then use a pasta machine to roll and cut it into strips.

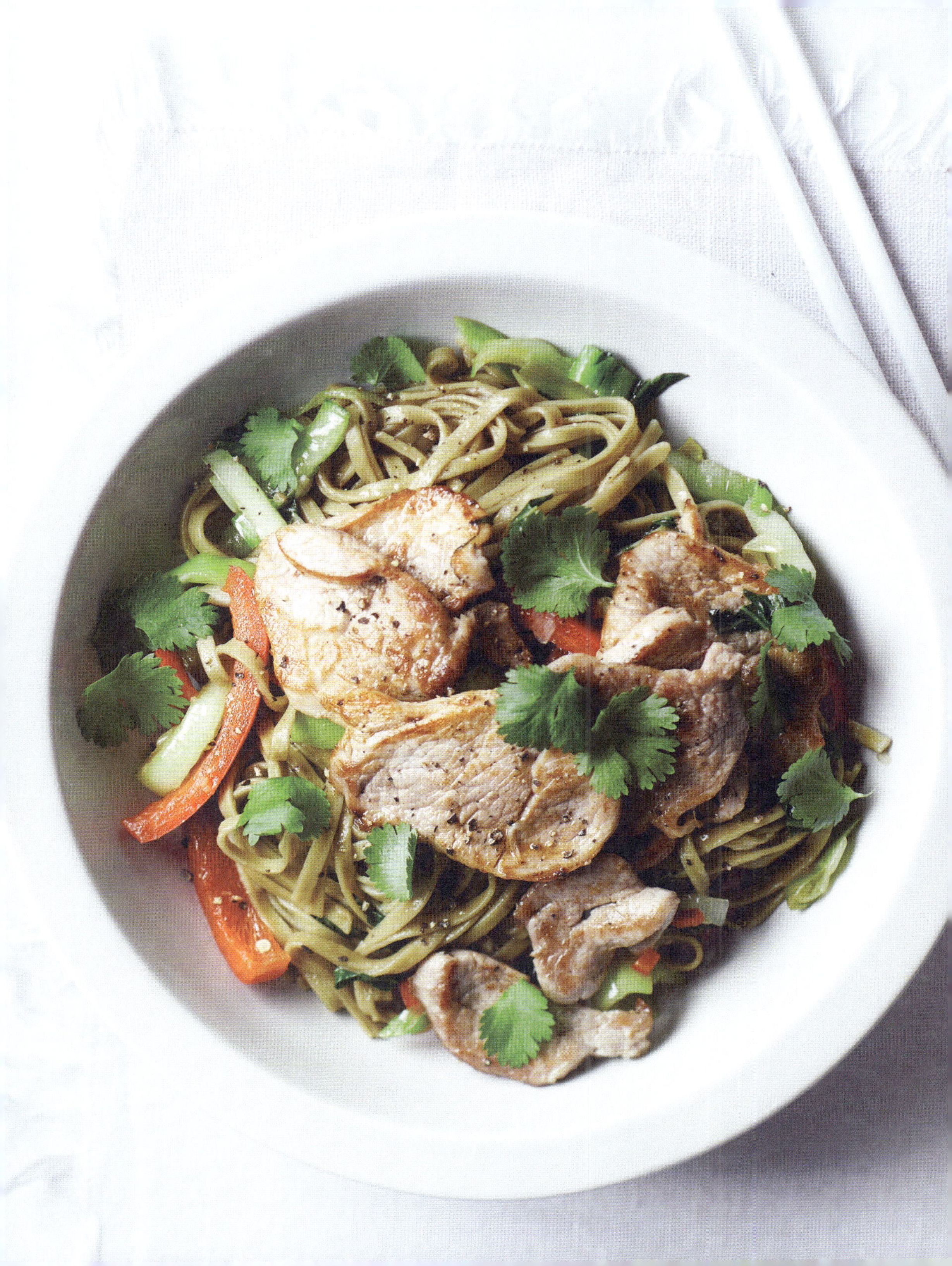

Bakes

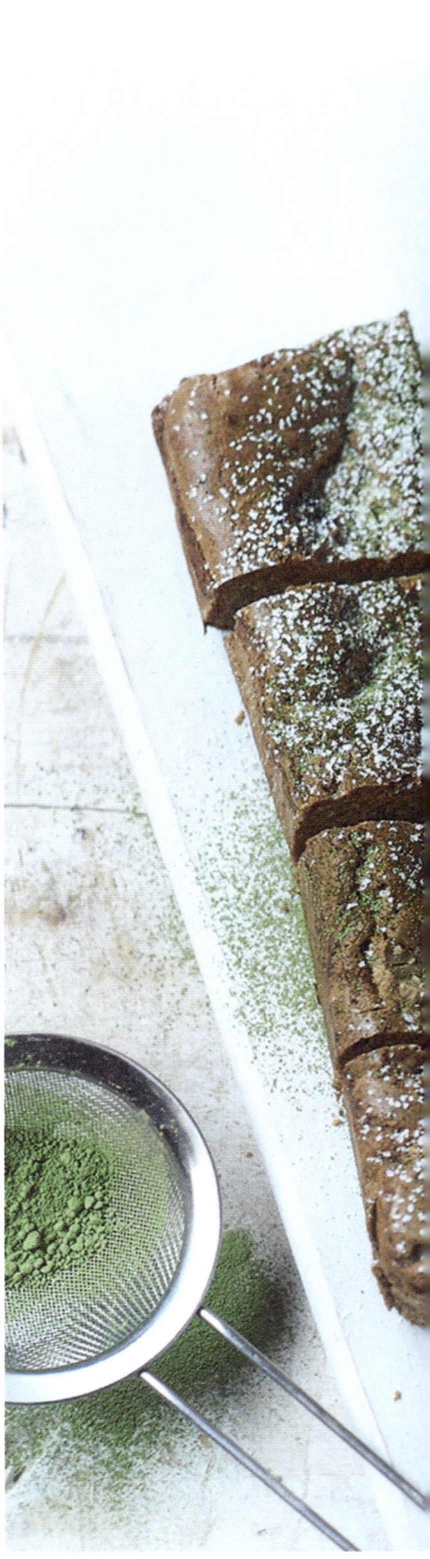

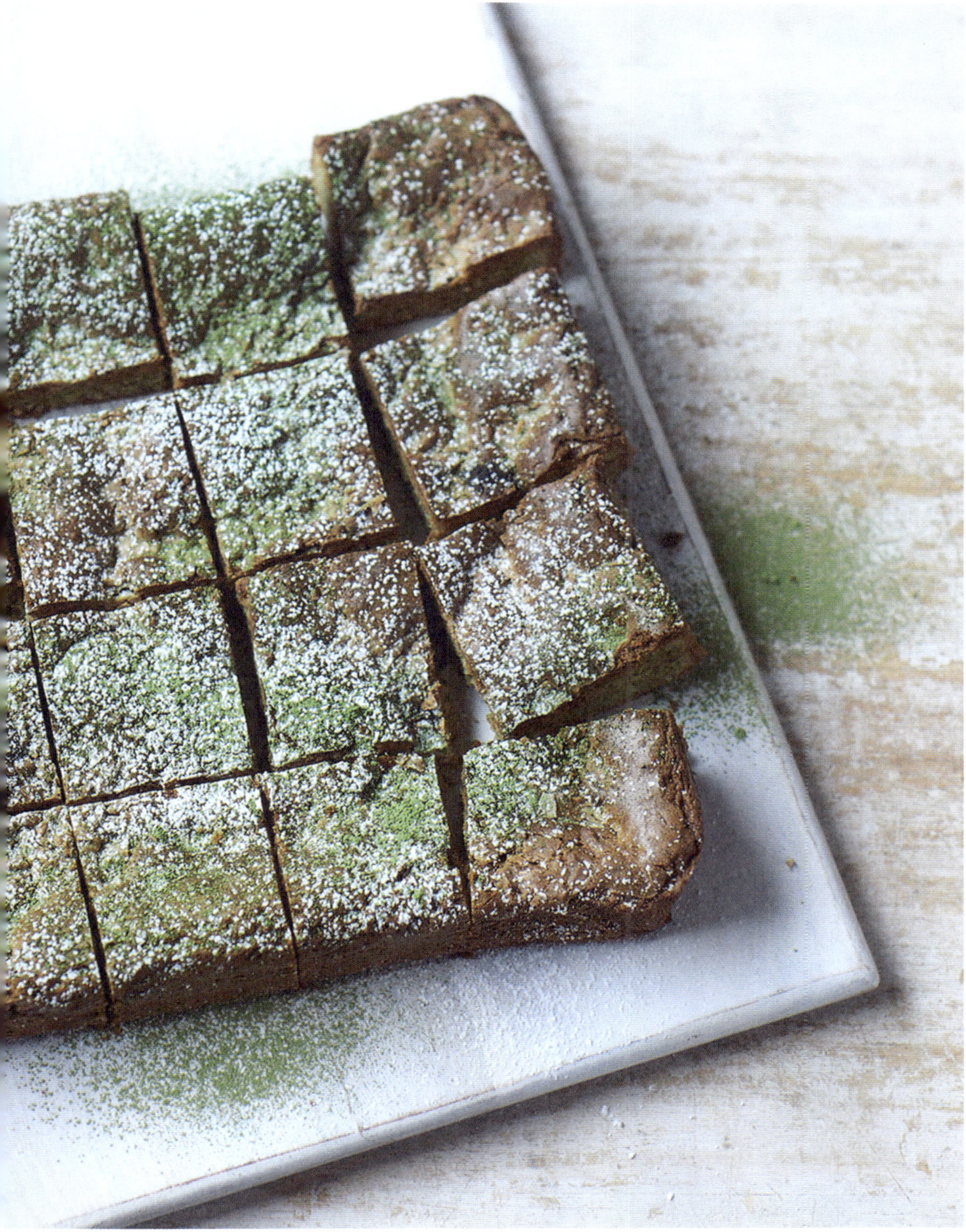

Chocolate layer cake with matcha icing

Wow, wow, wow! This is a truly impressive, truly indulgent celebration cake. Best enjoyed with a Matcha latte (see page 62), or even a Mint fizz cocktail (see page 70).

MAKES ONE 20CM/ 8IN CAKE

225g (1 cup) butter, plus extra for greasing
225g (1 cup) caster (superfine) sugar
4 eggs
175g (1½ cups) self-raising (rising) flour
60g (½ cup) cocoa powder
½ tsp baking powder
chocolate cake decorations (optional)

FOR THE MATCHA BUTTERCREAM ICING (FROSTING)

1 tbsp matcha powder
2 tbsp milk
225g (1 cup) unsalted butter, at room temperature
450g (4 cups) icing (confectioner's) sugar

1 Preheat the oven to 170°C fan/190°C/375°F/gas mark 5. Lightly butter two 20cm (8in) cake tins (pans) and line the bases with baking parchment.

2 Cream the butter and sugar in a food mixer or food processor until light and fluffy. Beat in the eggs, one at a time, adding a little flour with each one to prevent the mixture curdling.

3 Sift the remaining flour with the cocoa powder and baking powder and add to the mixture on a slow speed until thoroughly blended. If it seems too thick, you can thin it with a little milk.

4 Divide the mixture between the two lined cake tins and lightly smooth the top. Bake in the preheated oven for 20–25 minutes until well risen and the sponge is starting to come away from the sides of the tins. When you press it gently, it should spring back.

5 Leave to cool for 10 minutes, before turning out onto a wire rack. When cold, remove the lining paper.

6 Make the matcha buttercream icing: blend the matcha powder and milk in a small bowl until you have a smooth paste. In a food mixer or food processor, or with a hand-held electric whisk, beat the butter until soft and then gradually beat in the icing sugar with the matcha paste until the icing is thick and smooth.

7 Cut each cold cake in half horizontally with a long-bladed knife. Spread the icing over three of the sponges and sandwich them together. Top with the remaining sponge layer and cover with the rest of the icing, smoothing it with a (step-) palette knife.

8 Decorate the cake, if wished, with chocolate shards or curls.

VARIATION

- Try adding some chocolate chips to the cake mixture or 2 tbsp espresso.

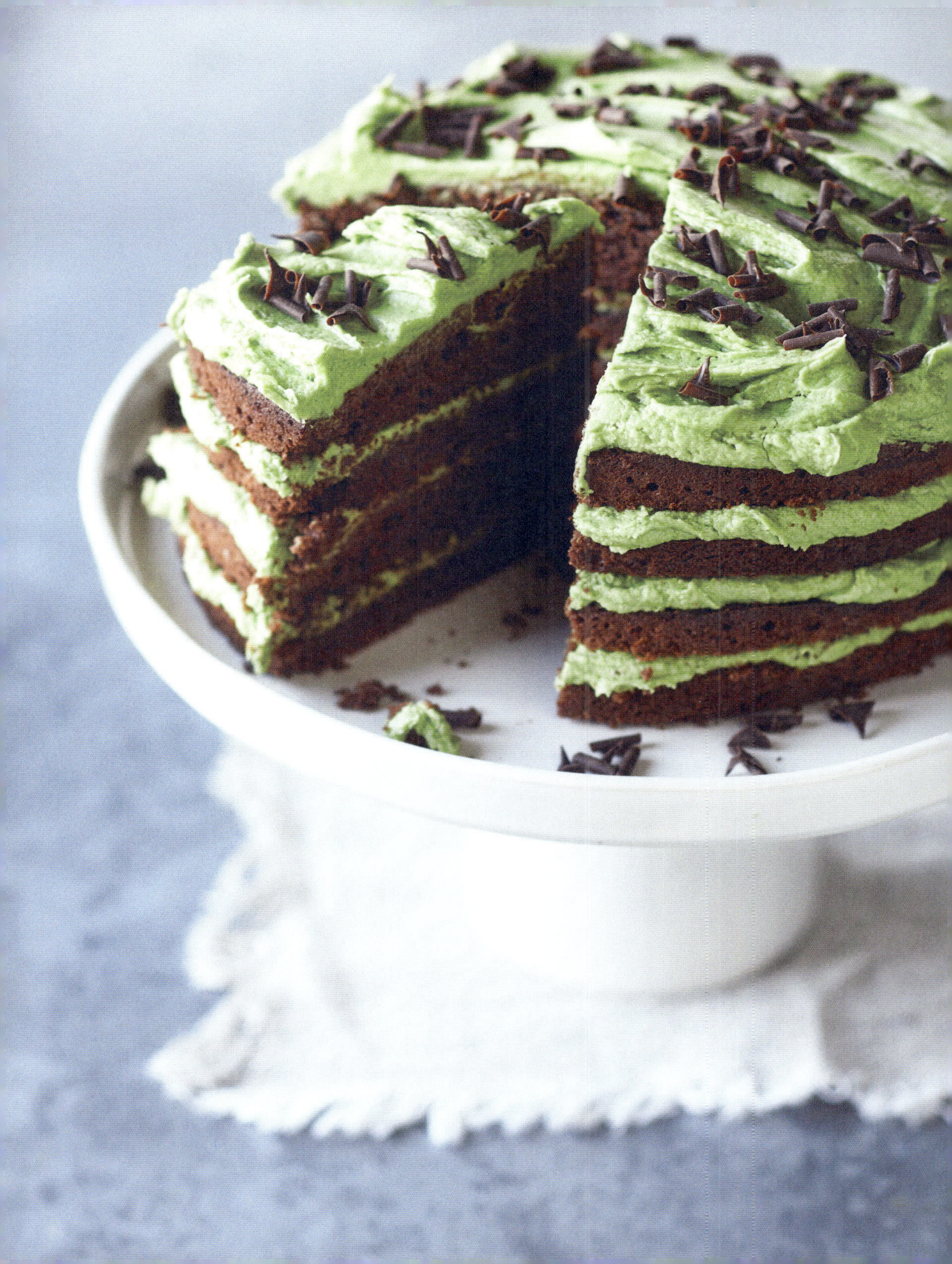

Matcha Swiss roll

The combination of matcha with this lemony filling is gorgeous. This is a lovely dessert with fresh strawberries or raspberries, or why not try orange rather than lemon curd?

SERVES 8

oil, for greasing
125g (½ cup) caster (superfine) sugar, plus extra for dusting
125g (1 cup) plus 2 tbsp plain (all-purpose) flour, plus extra for dusting
3 large eggs
1 tbsp matcha powder
1 tbsp lukewarm water

FOR THE CREAMY LEMON CURD FILLING
300ml (1¼ cups) double (heavy) cream
4 tbsp lemon curd

1 Preheat the oven to 180°C fan/200°C/400°F/gas mark 6. Lightly brush a 33 x 23cm (13 x 9in) Swiss roll tin (baking sheet) with oil and then line with baking parchment. Brush the paper with oil and then lightly dust with caster sugar and flour.

2 Put the eggs and sugar in a large mixing bowl and beat with a hand-held electric whisk until the mixture is pale and thick (about three times the original volume) and leaves a trail when you lift the whisk into the air. Be patient and don't take shortcuts as this step is key – you may have to keep whisking for 10 minutes to get to this stage.

3 Sift the flour into a clean bowl and gently stir in the matcha powder until thoroughly mixed. Tip half into the cake mixture and mix in gently but thoroughly, with a metal spoon, in a figure-of-eight movement. Repeat with the remaining flour. Fold in the water.

4 Pour the mixture into the prepared tin and spread it out evenly right into the corners. Bake in the preheated oven for 10–12 minutes until risen and firm to the touch.

5 Place a damp clean tea (kitchen) towel on the work surface and a large sheet of baking parchment on top. Dust the paper with sugar.

6 Loosen the warm sponge by running a knife around the edge and gently invert it onto the sugar-dusted paper. Carefully peel away the baking parchment and neatly trim the edges of the sponge. Cover with another sheet of baking parchment and roll it up gently from one of the short ends, using the paper and tea towel underneath to help you. Do not worry if it cracks a little – just roll it slowly and always use a damp tea towel underneath to help prevent cracking.

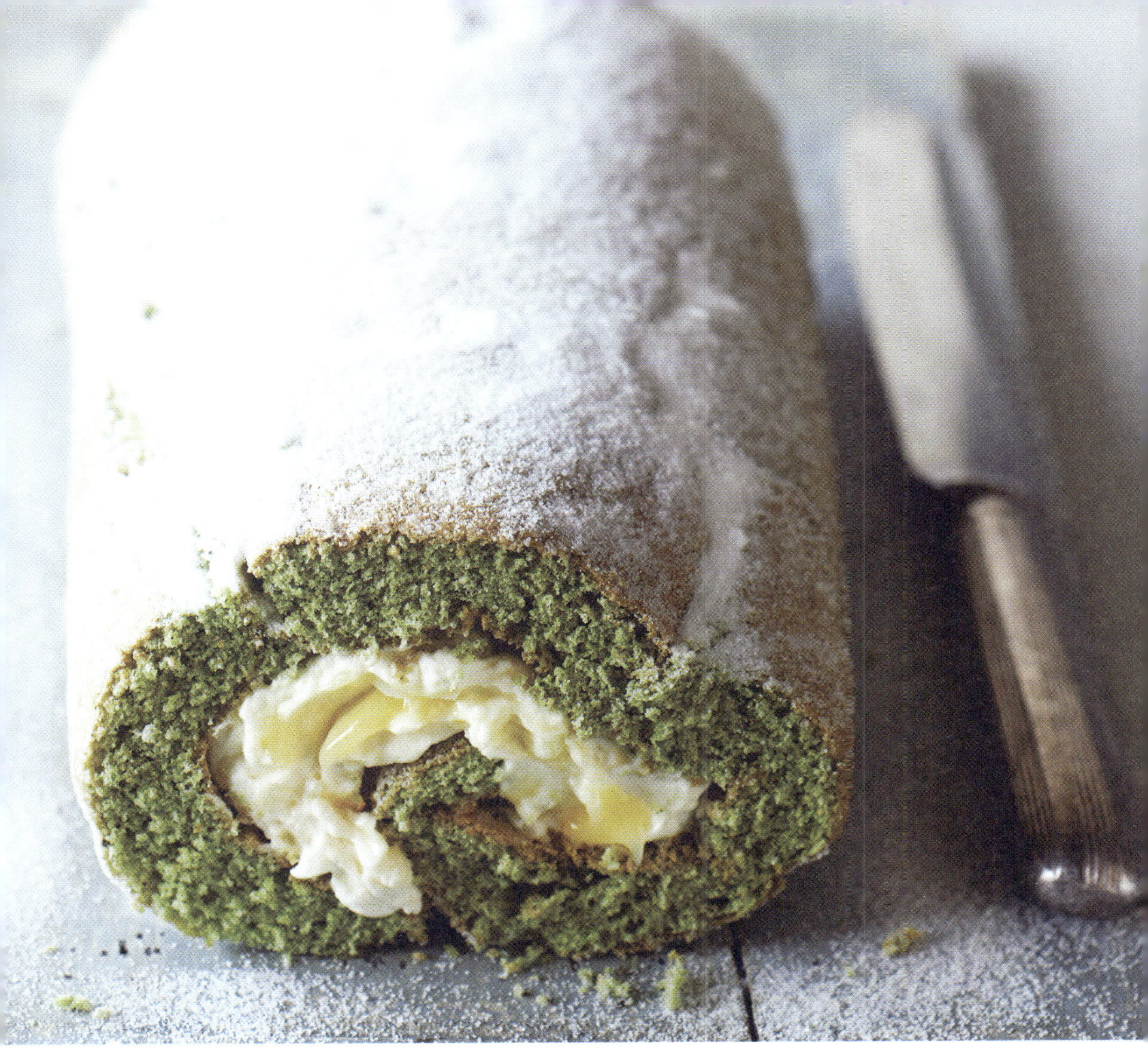

7 To make the filling, whip the cream in a clean bowl until thick. Gently swirl in the lemon curd to create a marbled effect.

8 When the sponge is cold, gently unroll it and spread with the filling, leaving a small border around the edge. Gently and slowly roll up the cake (be careful as it is prone to cracking) and place it, seam-side down, on a plate. Dust with sugar and serve cut into slices.

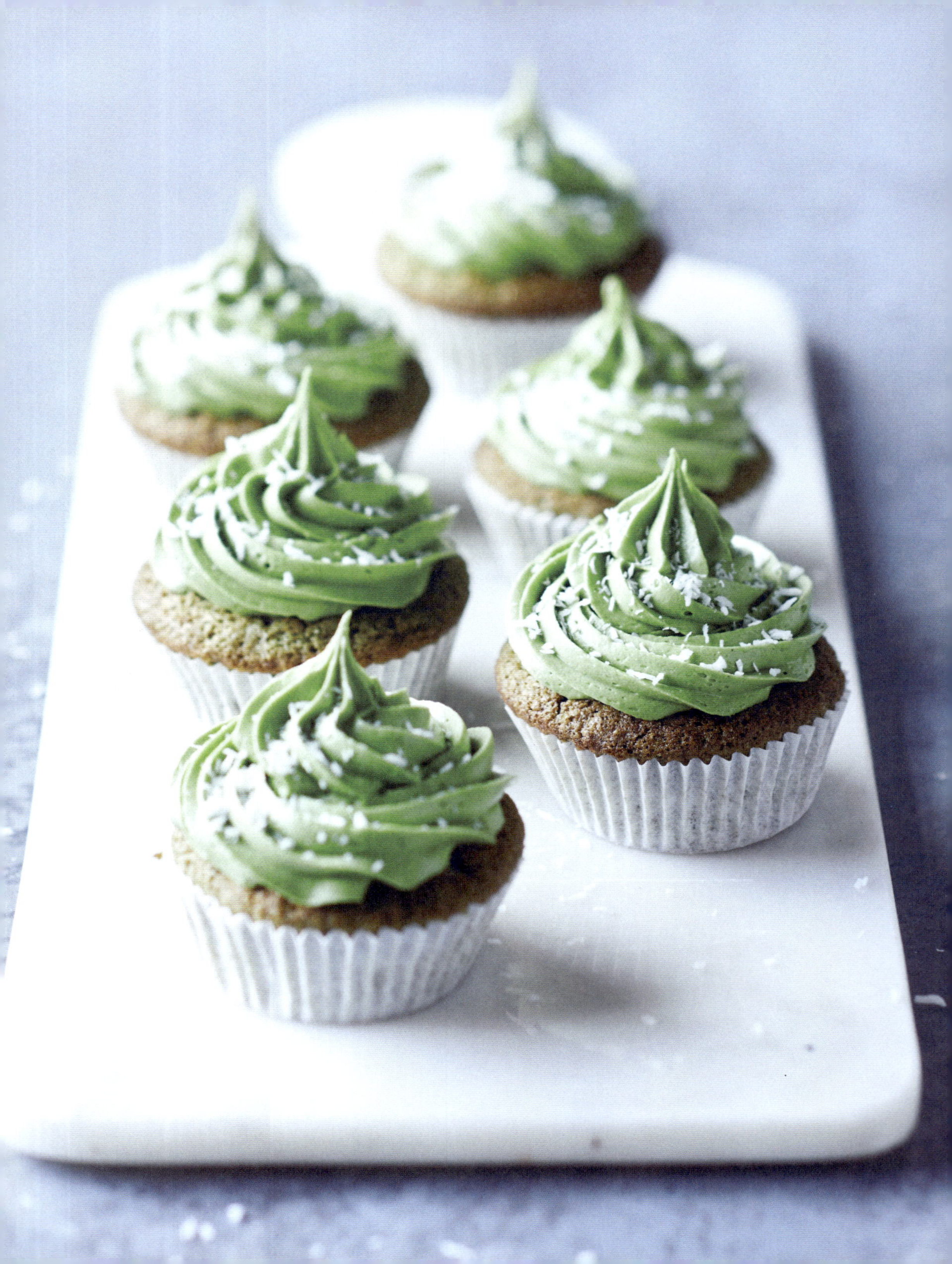

Coconut and matcha cupcakes

Coconut and matcha is one of our favourite combinations. These cupcakes are just divine – light and fluffy with a delicious coconut and matcha icing (frosting).

MAKES 12 CAKES

60g (½ stick) butter
175g (¾ cup) caster (superfine) sugar
1 large egg
125g (1 cup) plus 2 tbsp plain (all-purpose) flour
1 tsp baking powder
¼ tsp bicarbonate of (baking) soda
pinch of salt
1 tbsp matcha powder
120ml (½ cup) coconut milk
desiccated coconut, to decorate

FOR THE COCONUT MATCHA ICING (FROSTING)

250g (2 cups) icing (confectioner's) sugar
5 tbsp unsalted butter
1 tbsp matcha powder
2 tbsp coconut cream

1 Preheat the oven to 160°C fan/180°C/350°F/gas mark 4. Line a 12-hole muffin tin (pan) with paper cases (cupcake liners).

2 In an electric mixer or food processor, beat the butter and sugar until the mixture is light and fluffy. Add the egg and beat well.

3 Sift the flour, baking powder, bicarbonate of soda, salt and matcha powder into a clean bowl.

4 Gradually add the dry ingredients to the cake mixture, beating until well mixed. Beat in the coconut milk, a little at a time.

5 Divide the cake mixture between the paper cases and bake in the preheated oven for about 15–20 minutes, until the cakes are well risen and spring back when you press them lightly with a finger. Cool on a wire rack.

6 Meanwhile, make the coconut matcha icing. In an electric mixer or food processor, beat together the icing sugar, butter and matcha powder until well blended and creamy. On a slow speed, add the coconut cream and then beat on a higher speed until the icing is really fluffy. This may take a few minutes. Alternatively, make this in a large bowl with a hand-held electric whisk.

7 When the cakes have cooled completely, decorate them with the icing and sprinkle with desiccated coconut. They will stay fresh for 3 days if stored in an airtight container.

VARIATIONS

- You can omit the matcha powder from the icing and lightly sprinkle a little over the tops of the decorated cakes instead of coconut.
- Add the grated zest and juice of a lime to the cake mixture and sprinkle some finely shredded lime zest over the icing.

Matcha blondies

These moreish matcha blondies are a Friday afternoon treat in the teapigs' office. We hope you will love them just as much as we do!

MAKES ABOUT 12 BLONDIES

200g (1 cup) butter
200g (7oz) white chocolate, chopped
250g (1 cup) soft brown sugar or muscovado sugar
3 eggs
200g (2 cups) self-raising (rising) flour
pinch of salt
1 tsp vanilla extract
3 tsp matcha powder, plus extra for dusting
icing (confectioner's) sugar, for dusting

1 Preheat the oven to 160°C fan/180°C/350°F/gas mark 4. Line the base of a 25 x 25cm (10 x 10in) cake tin (brownie pan) with baking parchment.

2 Melt the butter in a saucepan and cook it very gently over a low heat for about 5 minutes until it turns golden.

3 Take the saucepan off the heat, add half the white chocolate and stir until smooth. Leave to cool.

4 In a large bowl, beat the sugar and eggs together until pale and fluffy. Add the flour, salt, vanilla, matcha powder and the cooled chocolate-butter mixture and fold it all in gently until it's evenly mixed.

5 Pour the mixture into the tin then scatter the rest of the white chocolate over the top of the mix. Bake for 40 minutes or until risen all over. Leave to cool, then dust with a little matcha powder and icing sugar. Delicious!

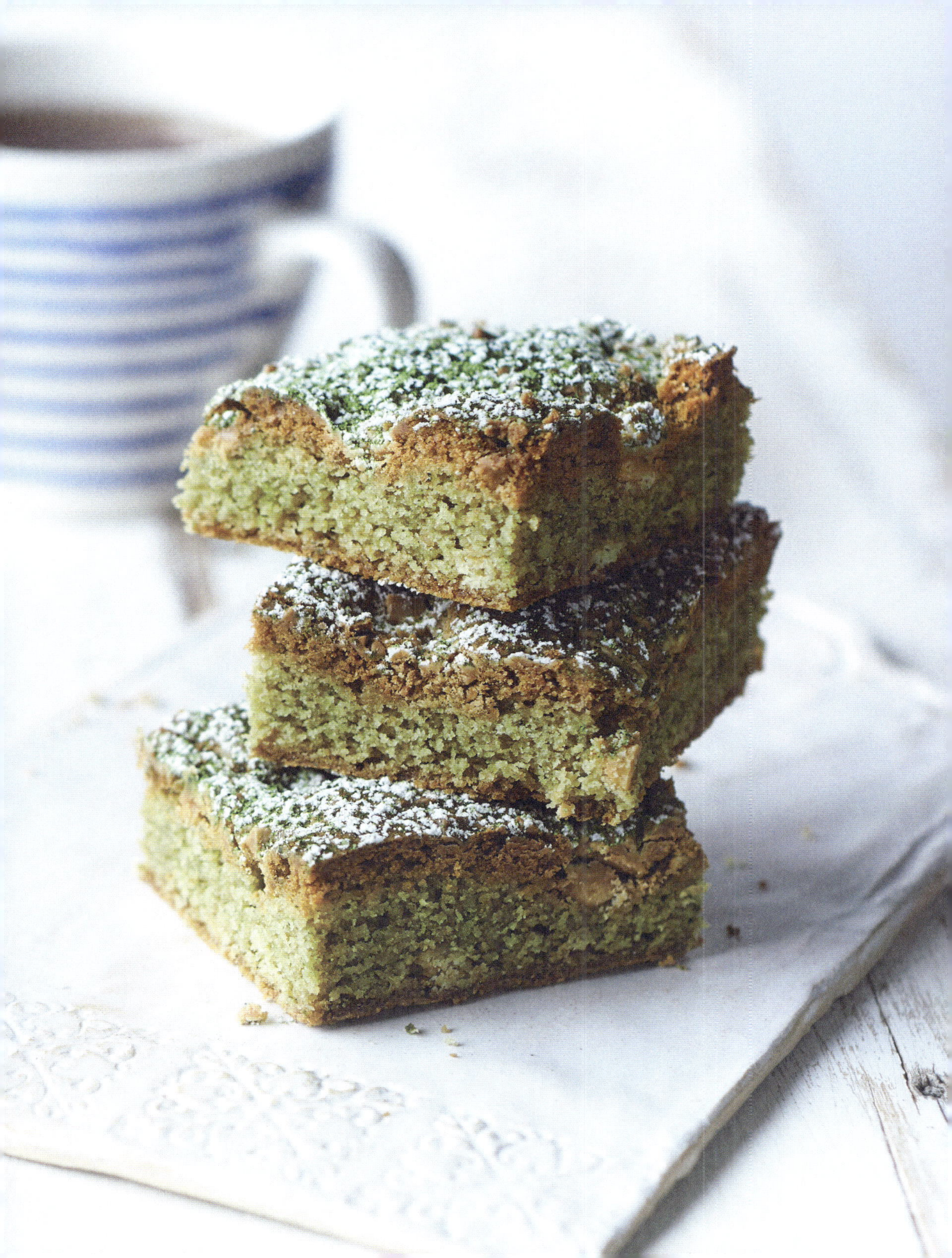

Matcha ring doughnuts

These doughnuts are really fun to make. Once you have got the hang of the recipe, why not experiment with different spices like nutmeg or cinnamon.

MAKES ABOUT 12 DOUGHNUTS

300g (2½ cups) plain (all-purpose) flour, plus extra for dusting
2 tsp matcha powder
3 tsp baking powder
½ tsp bicarbonate of (baking) soda
½ tsp salt
60g (¼ cup) granulated sugar
1 large egg
150ml (½ cup) buttermilk
2 tbsp butter, melted
vegetable oil, for deep-frying

FOR THE MATCHA GLAZE
250g (2 cups) icing (confectioner's) sugar
1 tbsp matcha powder
1 egg white
1 tbsp water

1 To make the matcha glaze, sift the icing sugar into a bowl and stir in the matcha powder. Add the egg white and water and whisk everything together until well combined. Set aside while you make the doughnuts.

2 Put the flour, matcha powder, baking powder, bicarbonate of soda, salt and sugar in a large bowl and mix together. Make a well in the centre.

3 In a separate bowl, beat together the egg, buttermilk and melted butter. Pour into the flour mixture and stir well until it forms a sticky dough.

4 Turn the dough out onto a floured work surface and roll it out or pat it down with your hands to a thickness of 1cm (½in). Cut into rounds with an 8cm (3in) pastry cutter. Use a smaller cutter, about 2.5cm (1in), to make a hole in the centre of each round. Roll out the leftover dough to make more doughnuts.

5 Meanwhile, pour some vegetable oil into a deep, heavy-based saucepan to a depth of 10cm (4in) and place over a medium heat. When it reaches 180°C/350°F on a sugar (candy) thermometer, you can start frying the doughnuts.

6 Fry the doughnuts in batches, three at a time, for about 3 minutes until golden, turning them halfway through. Remove and drain on kitchen paper (paper towels).

7 Dip the warm doughnuts in the matcha glaze and eat them while they're fresh and still warm.

VARIATION

- Instead of a glaze, try dipping the warm doughnuts in a sifted and combined mixture of icing sugar and matcha powder. You will need 1 tbsp matcha powder and 125g (1 cup) icing sugar.

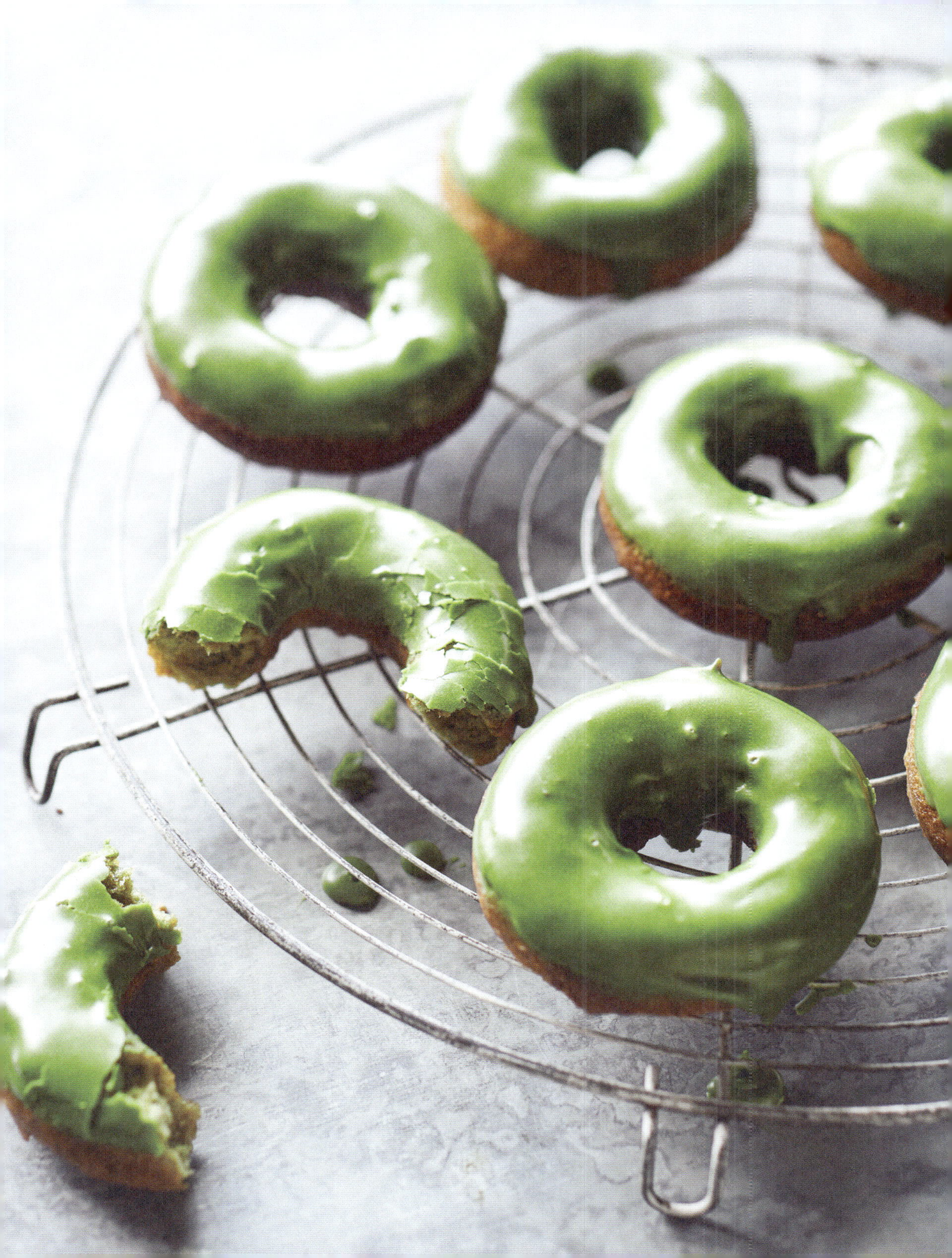

Matcha macarons

These macarons are truly delicious – matcha works so well with almonds. These delicate and sweet little treats look very cool and amazingly green!

MAKES ABOUT 30 MACARONS

175g (1½ cups) icing (confectioner's) sugar
175g (1 cup) ground almonds
1 tsp matcha powder
4 egg whites, divided
175g (¾ cup) granulated sugar
50ml (¼ cup) water
a few drops green food colouring (optional)

FOR THE MATCHA BUTTERCREAM

125g (1 stick) unsalted butter
125g (1 cup) icing (confectioner's) sugar
1 tbsp matcha powder
1 tbsp milk

1 Put the icing sugar, ground almonds and matcha powder in a food processor and pulse until well mixed and finely ground. Sift into a large mixing bowl and if any particles are left in the sieve, pulse and sift them again.

2 Add 2 egg whites and mix with a wooden spoon until you have a thick paste.

3 Put the remaining 2 egg whites in a clean heatproof bowl. Set aside while you make the sugar syrup.

4 To make the sugar syrup, put the granulated sugar and water in a small saucepan over a medium-high heat. Stir to dissolve the sugar and bring to the boil. Cook the syrup until it reaches 110°C/225°F on a sugar (candy) thermometer.

5 Immediately start beating the egg whites with an electric whisk on the high setting. As soon as the syrup reaches 118°C/239°F remove from the heat and pour it in a thin stream into the egg whites, whisking all the time on a high speed until the meringue looks glossy with stiff peaks and cools slightly.

6 Gently fold half of the meringue into the matcha almond mixture with a spatula, taking care not to over-mix it. Fold in the remaining meringue and 2–3 drops of food colouring (if using). Add this very carefully, a drop at a time, until you have the required pale green. Keep folding the meringue and matcha mixture until it's really smooth, evenly coloured, and if you lift the spatula it falls in a ribbon and blends back into the mixture without a trace.

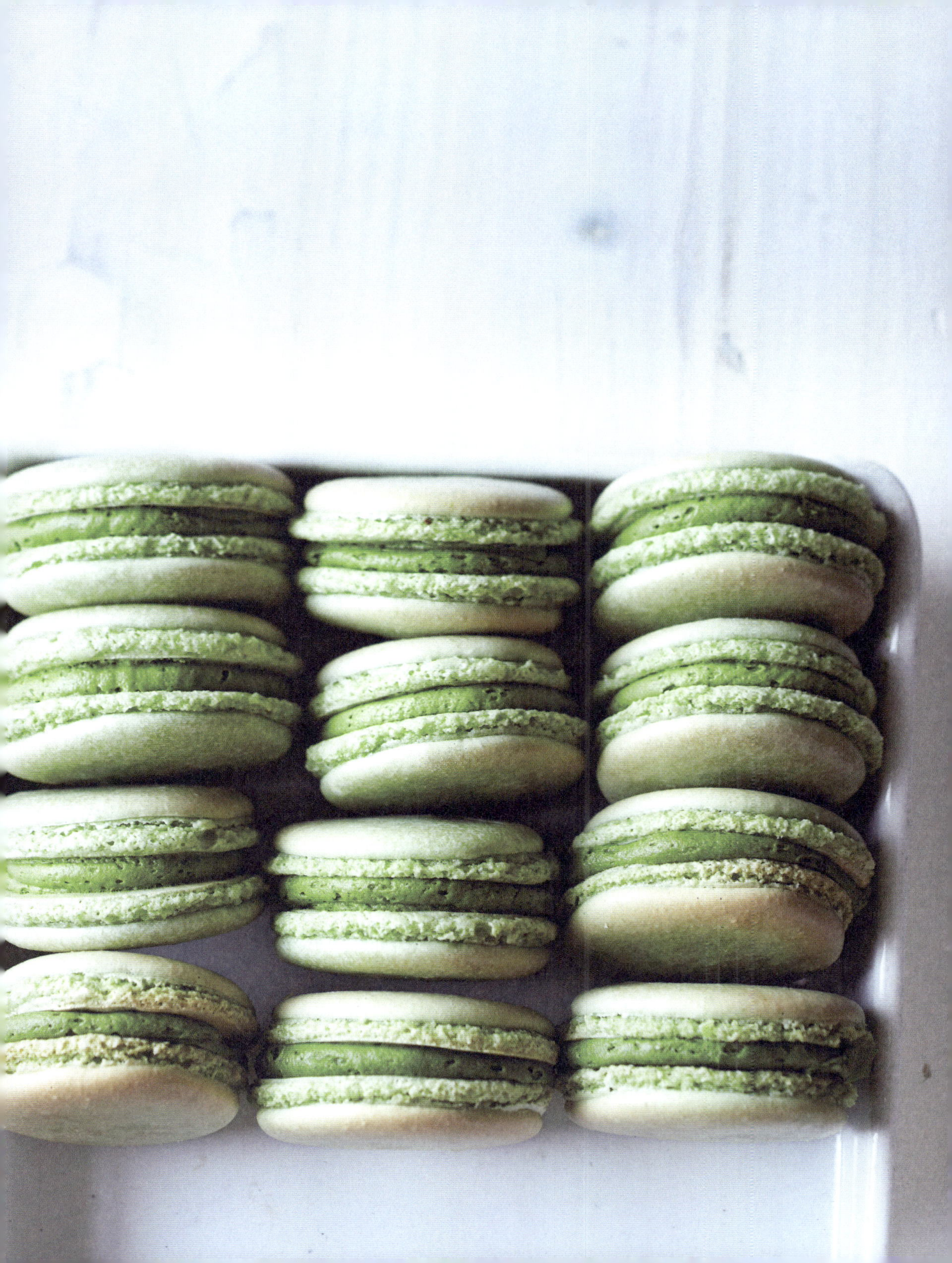

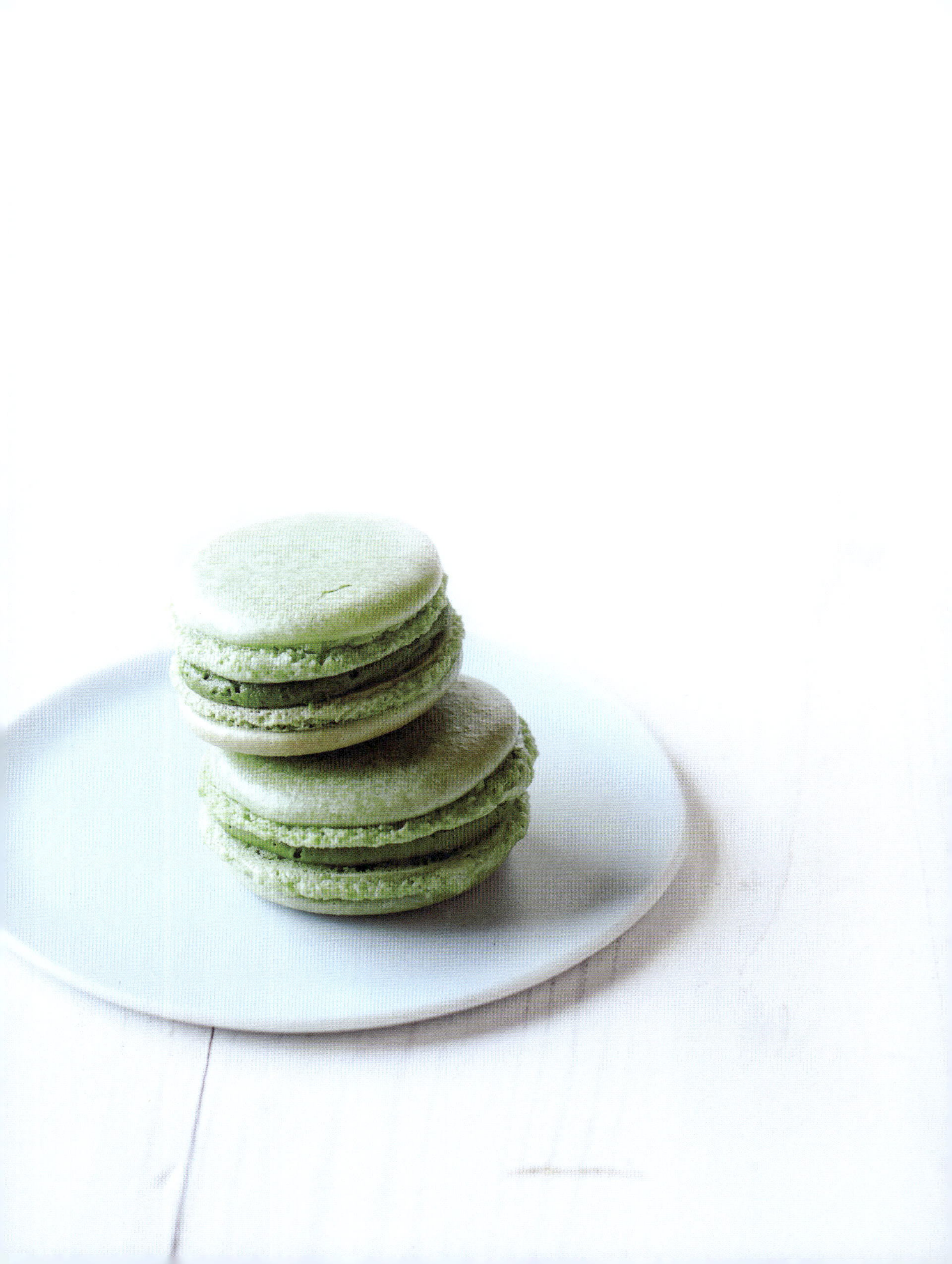

7 Line 2 baking trays (sheets) with baking parchment.

8 Spoon the meringue mixture into a piping (pastry) bag fitted with a wide plain nozzle (round tip) and pipe circles of 3.5cm (1½in) diameter on to the baking parchment until all the mixture is used up. Set aside to rest for 30 minutes and preheat the oven to 150°C fan/170°C/325°F/gas mark 3.

9 Bake the macarons in the preheated oven for 12–14 minutes until set. Keep checking after 12 minutes to make sure they don't brown. Carefully slide the baking parchment off the baking trays onto a cool surface and leave to cool. Then peel off the baking parchment.

10 To make the matcha buttercream filling, whisk the butter until fluffy in a food mixer and then beat in the icing sugar and matcha powder. Add the milk and whisk until thick and smooth.

11 Use the buttercream to sandwich the macarons together. You can smear it on with a teaspoon but it looks neater piped on.

12 Store the macarons in an airtight container in the fridge.

Raisin, oat and matcha cookies

These irresistible crispy cookies are perfect for sharing when you have friends over for a cup of matcha! No need for guilt when you take your second or third . . .

MAKES ABOUT 30 COOKIES

125g (1 cup) raisins
200g (1 cup) butter
200g (1 cup) soft brown sugar
2 large eggs
1 tsp vanilla extract
125g (1¼ cups) rolled oats
275g (2½ cups) plain (all-purpose) flour, sifted
1½ tsp matcha powder
1 tsp bicarbonate of (baking) soda
1 tsp ground cinnamon
½ tsp grated nutmeg
pinch of salt

1 Preheat the oven to 160°C fan/180°C/350°F/gas mark 4. Line two baking trays (sheets) with baking parchment.

2 Put the raisins in a bowl and cover with boiling water. Set aside to soak for 20–30 minutes – they will swell and become plump. Drain and reserve the soaking liquid.

3 In a food mixer or using a hand-held electric whisk, beat the butter and sugar until pale, light and fluffy. Beat in the eggs, one a time, and then the vanilla.

4 Add the oats, flour, matcha powder, bicarbonate of soda, cinnamon, nutmeg, salt and raisins. Mix to a soft dough, adding some of the reserved soaking liquid or a little milk if the mixture is too dry.

5 Using a tablespoon, drop spoonfuls of the mixture onto the lined baking trays and flatten slightly with your hand. Make sure there's plenty of space between them as they will spread out during cooking.

6 Bake in the preheated oven for 12–15 minutes until golden brown. Leave to cool on the trays or transfer to a wire rack. Store in an airtight container.

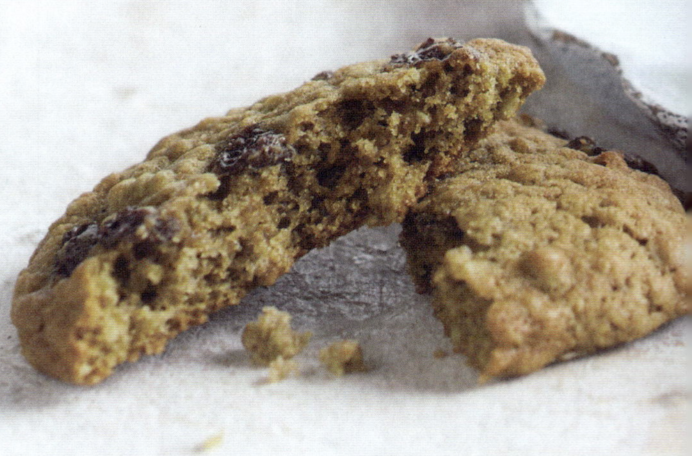

VARIATIONS

- For neater cookies, chill the dough in the fridge for 30 minutes before rolling it out and cutting it with a cookie cutter. Bake as as per page 148.
- Substitute dried cranberries, cherries or blueberries for the raisins. There's no need to soak them.
- For extra texture, add 2–3 tbsp of sunflower seeds to the mix.

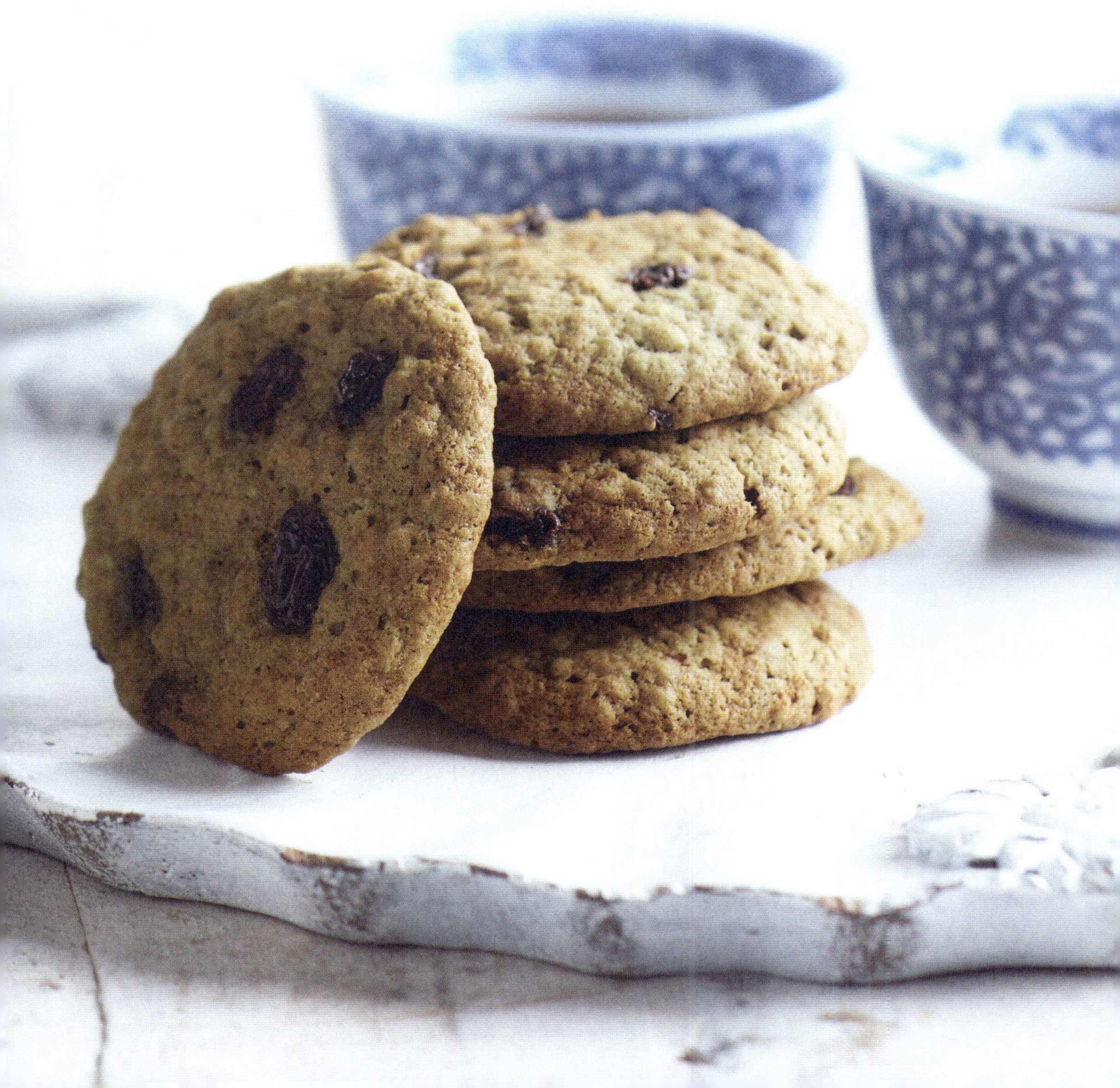

Desserts

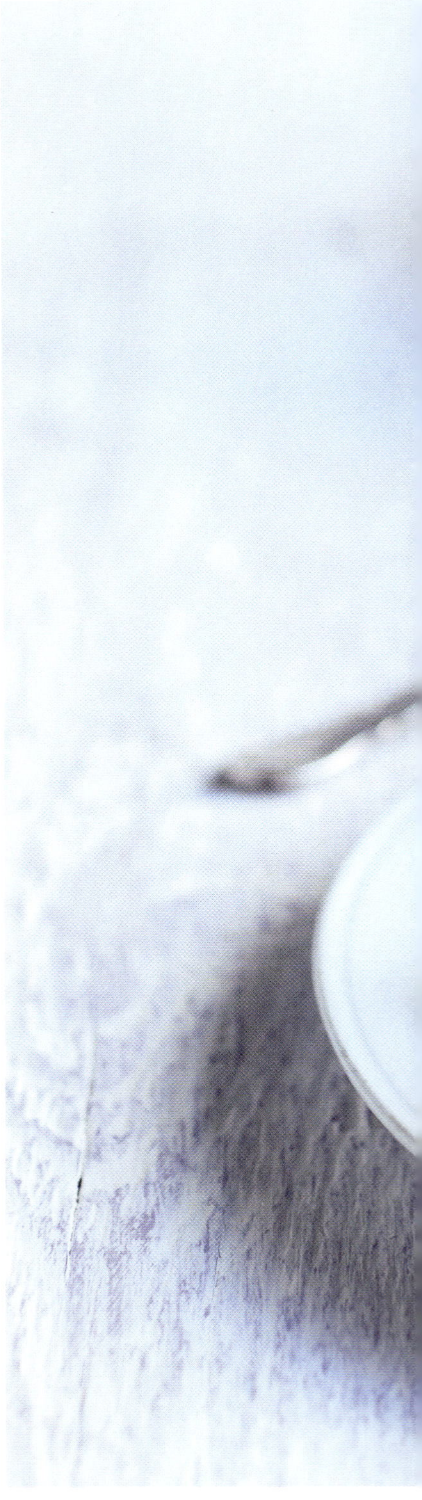

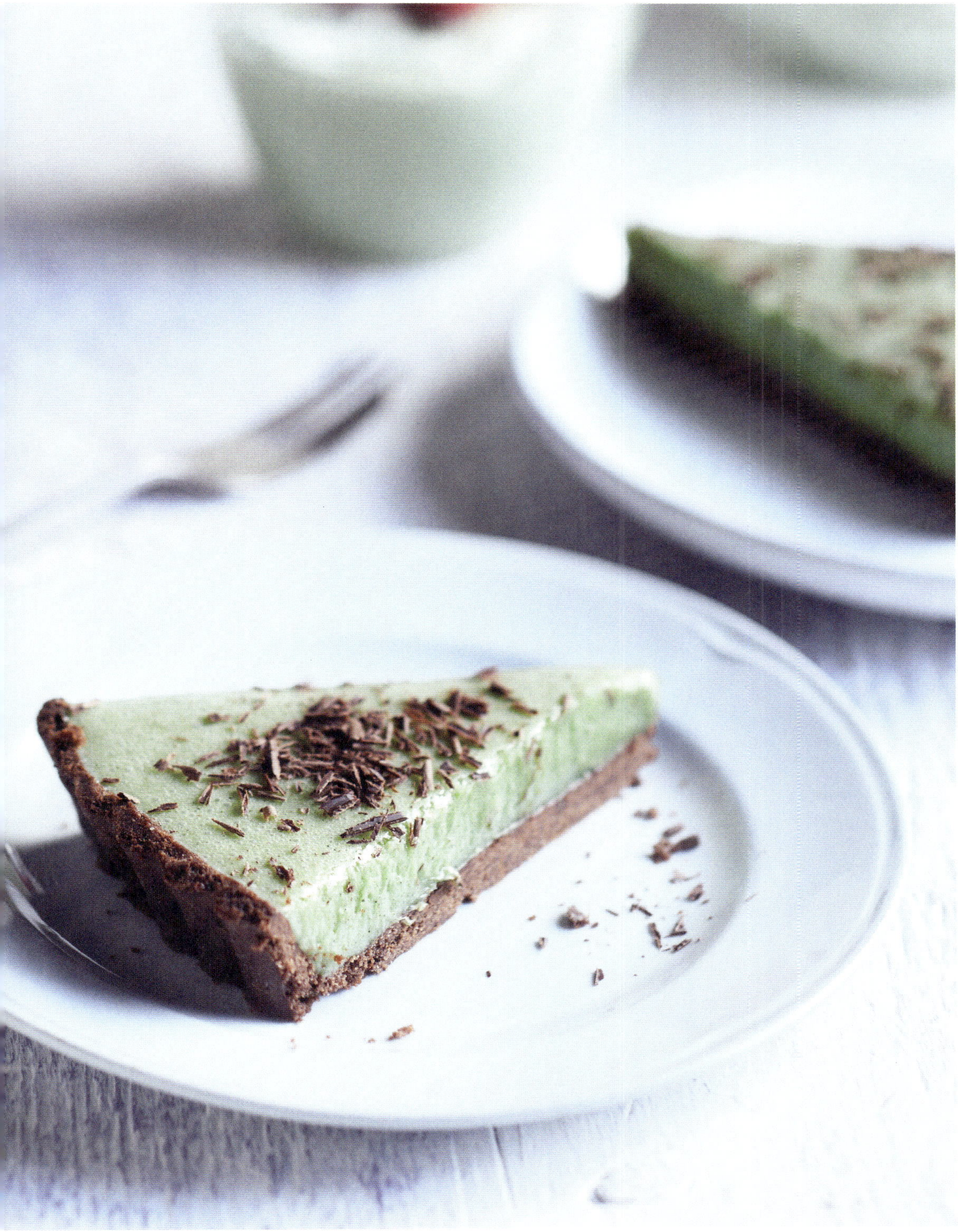

Matcha soufflés

These beautifully light, vibrant green soufflés are real showstoppers. If you would rather make a single large soufflé, simply bake for a little longer – about 25–30 minutes.

SERVES 4

melted butter for greasing
60g (¼ cup) caster (superfine) sugar, plus extra for coating
100ml (½ cup) double (heavy) cream
1 rounded tbsp plain (all-purpose) flour
3 rounded tsp cornflour (cornstarch)
1 tbsp matcha powder
125ml (½ cup) milk
2 egg yolks
4 egg whites
icing (confectioner's) sugar, for dusting

1 Preheat the oven to 160°C fan/180°C/350°F/gas mark 4. Brush the insides of four large ramekin dishes with melted butter and then lightly coat with caster sugar. Chill in the fridge while you make the soufflés.

2 Stir the cream, flour, cornflour and matcha powder together in a large bowl and whisk until smooth and no clumps remain.

3 Heat the milk in a large saucepan over a medium heat. As soon as it starts to boil, remove from the heat and immediately start whisking it, a little at a time, into the matcha mixture until smooth.

4 Return the mixture to the saucepan and beat continuously over a low heat until thick and smooth. Use a hand-held electric whisk to make this easier.

5 Beat the egg yolks and caster sugar together in a bowl until thick and then beat them into the matcha mixture, taking the saucepan off the heat to do so. Return the saucepan to the heat and keep whisking until you have a thick custard. Set aside to cool.

6 Meanwhile, beat the egg whites in a clean, dry bowl until soft peaks form. Gently fold them into the cooled matcha custard, using a spatula or large metal spoon.

7 When the mixture is evenly coloured throughout, divide it between the chilled ramekins, filling them right up to the top. Level the surface of each soufflé and gently run a (step-) palette knife or your thumbnail around the edge.

8 Place the ramekins on a baking tray (sheet) and cook in the preheated oven for 10–12 minutes until well risen and just starting to colour on top. Dust lightly with icing sugar and serve immediately.

VARIATION

- Instead of coating the insides of the ramekins with sugar you could use grated dark (bittersweet) chocolate.

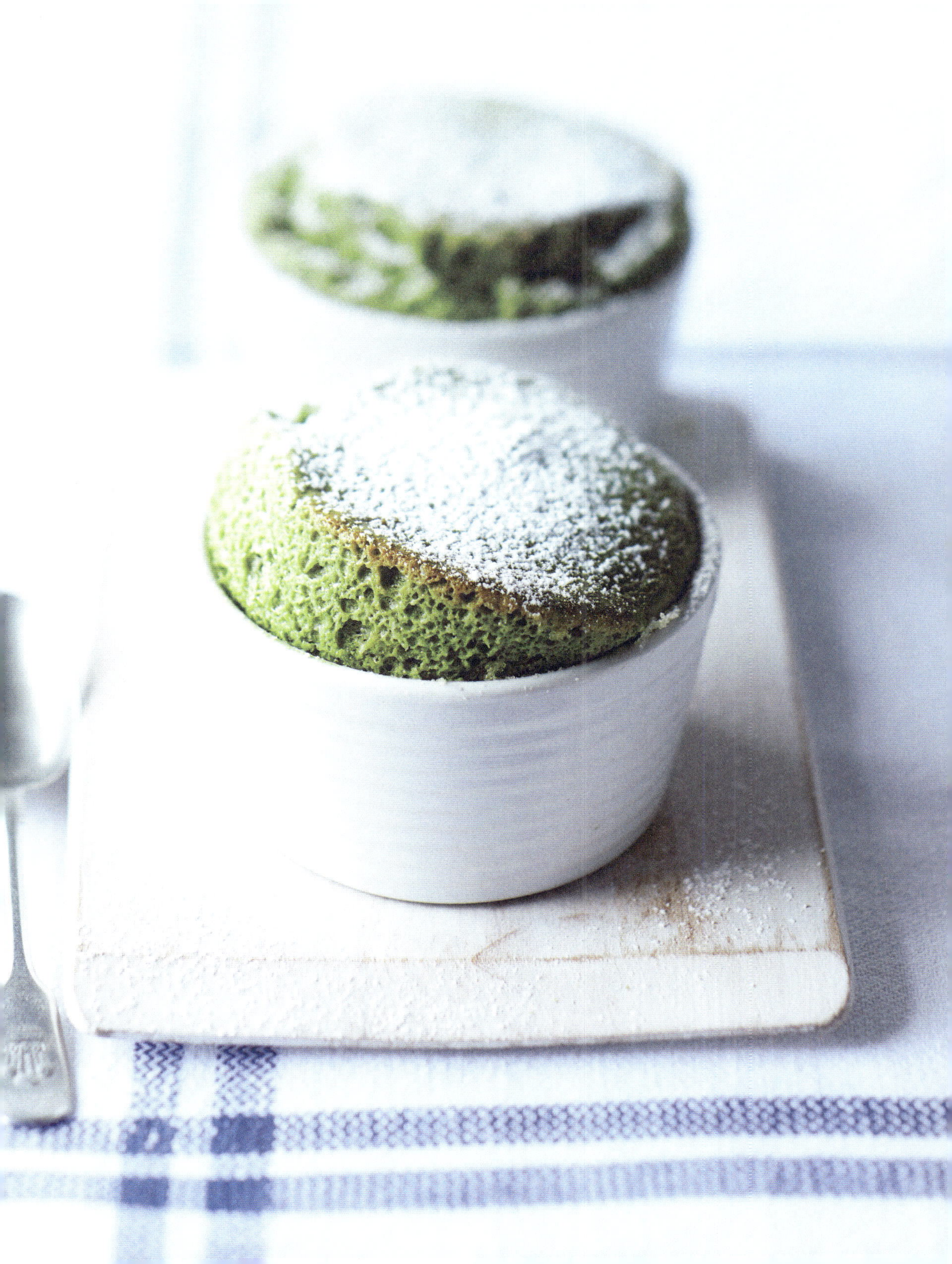

Mini matcha cheesecakes

Try using your favourite biscuits to make the base – Oreos (without the filling), digestives (graham crackers) or oat biscuits all work particularly well.

MAKES 4 MINI CHEESECAKES

250g (1 cup) cream cheese
1 tsp vanilla extract
4 tbsp caster (superfine) sugar
1 tbsp matcha powder, plus extra for sprinkling
5 tbsp warm water
4 sheets leaf gelatine
350ml (1½ cups) double (heavy) cream

FOR THE CHEESECAKE BASE

3 tbsp butter
1 tbsp golden (corn) syrup
150g (5oz) gingernut (gingersnap) biscuits

1 To make the cheesecake base, melt the butter with the golden syrup in a saucepan over a low heat. Blitz the biscuits to crumbs in a food processor and stir into the melted butter.

2 Divide the mixture between four large ramekins or four 10cm (4in) ring moulds placed on a baking tray (sheet) lined with baking parchment. Press down firmly with the back of a spoon to level.

3 In a bowl, beat the cream cheese with the vanilla and sugar.

4 Stir the matcha powder into the warm water, whisking until well mixed with no lumps.

5 Put the gelatine sheets in a dish of cold water and leave to soak for 5 minutes until softened, then remove and squeeze out any excess water.

6 Heat 100ml (½ cup) of the cream in a small saucepan over a low heat. When it's warm, remove from the heat and stir the gelatine into the cream until it dissolves.

7 Stir the cream mixture into the cream cheese mixture with the matcha until well mixed. Chill in the fridge for about 10 minutes until it begins to set.

8 Meanwhile, whip the rest of the cream in a clean mixing bowl until it forms soft peaks. Fold gently into the cream cheese mixture with a spatula or metal spoon.

9 Divide between the moulds or ramekin dishes and smooth the tops with a (step-) palette knife. Chill in the fridge for at least 4 hours until thoroughly set.

10 Serve in the ramekins or turn the mini cheesecakes out of the moulds by gently running a knife around the edge. Decorate by sprinkling with a little matcha powder.

VARIATIONS

- Instead of vanilla extract, flavour the cheesecake with some grated lime or lemon zest.
- You can also decorate the tops with chocolate curls or fresh fruit.

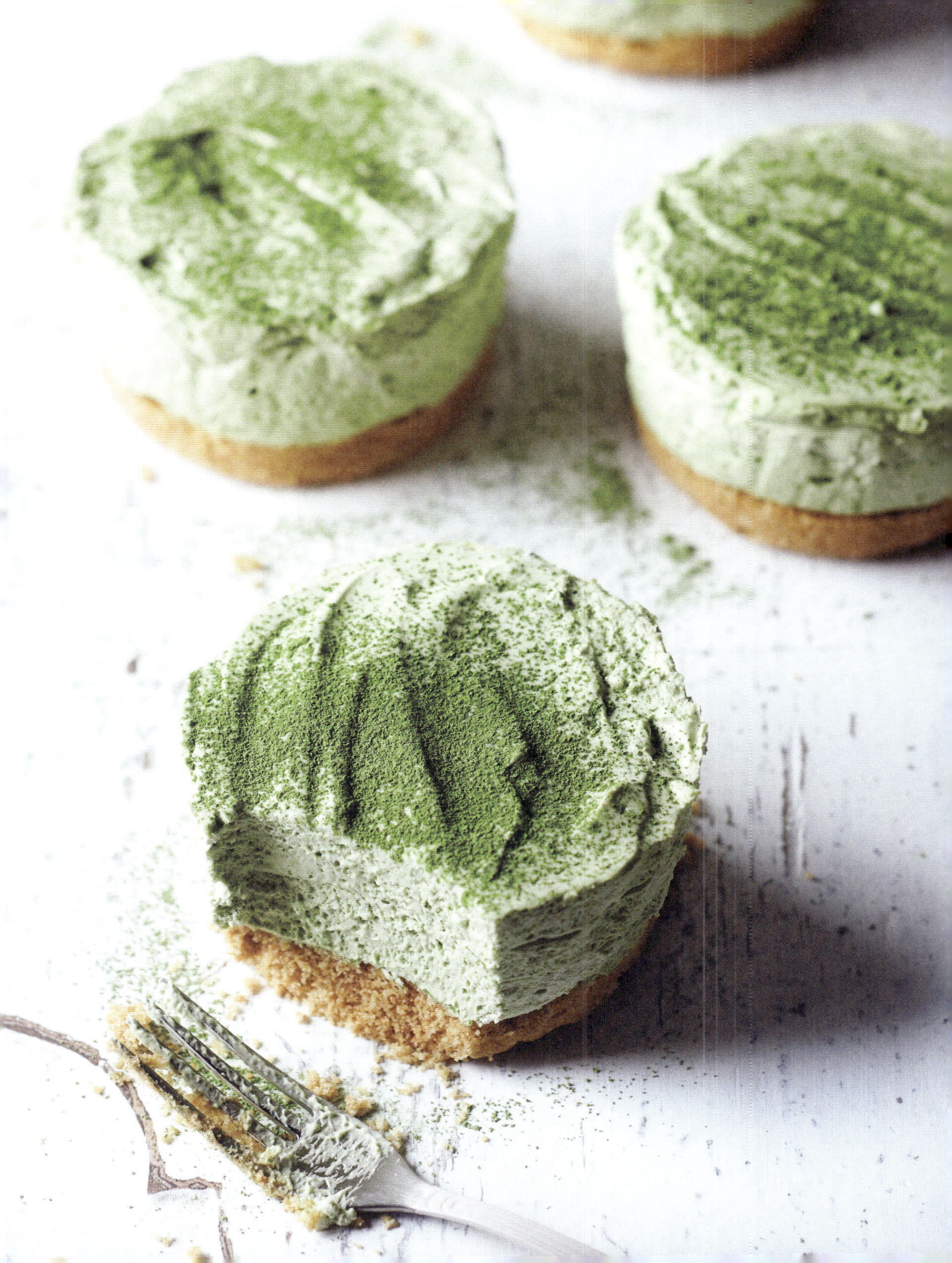

Chocolate and matcha tart

This tart is stunning dressed with chocolate shards or shavings. Try it served with fresh raspberries or strawberries and crème fraîche.

SERVES 8–10

400g (14oz) white chocolate, roughly chopped
300ml (1¼ cups) double (heavy) cream
few drops of vanilla extract
1 tbsp matcha powder
chocolate shavings, to decorate

FOR THE CHOCOLATE PASTRY (PIE SHELL)
175g (1½ cups) plain (all-purpose) flour, plus extra for dusting
40g (½ cup) cocoa powder
85g (⅔ cup) icing (confectioner's) sugar
150g (1¼ sticks) butter, cut into small pieces, plus extra for greasing
2 egg yolks

1 To make the chocolate pastry, sift the flour, cocoa powder and icing sugar into a large bowl. Rub in the butter with your fingertips until the mixture resembles breadcrumbs. Stir in the egg yolks until you have a soft dough. If it's too dry and crumbly, add a little cold water, 1 tbsp at a time.

2 Put the dough in a plastic bag or wrap in cling film (plastic wrap) and chill in the fridge for at least 30 minutes.

3 Preheat the oven to 150°C fan/170°C/325°F/gas mark 3. Roll out the dough on a lightly floured surface. Gently transfer to a lightly greased 23cm (9in) loose-bottomed tart tin (pan). Line with a sheet of baking parchment and fill with baking beans. Place on a baking tray (sheet).

4 Bake the tart 'blind' in the preheated oven for 20–25 minutes. Remove the baking parchment and beans and pop back into the oven for 10–15 minutes until the pastry is cooked and crisp. Set aside to cool.

5 To make the filling, melt the white chocolate in a heatproof bowl placed over a saucepan of gently simmering water, then remove from the heat.

6 Heat the cream in a small saucepan until it starts to boil. Beat into the melted chocolate with the vanilla extract and matcha powder, whisking until there are no lumps and the mixture is evenly coloured.

7 Pour the chocolate mixture into the pastry case and allow to cool a little. Chill in the fridge for at least 2 hours until set before turning out the tart onto a plate and sprinkling with chocolate shavings to serve.

VARIATION

- If you prefer, make a biscuit base with crushed Bourbons or Oreos, melted butter and melted dark (bittersweet) chocolate (see page 154).

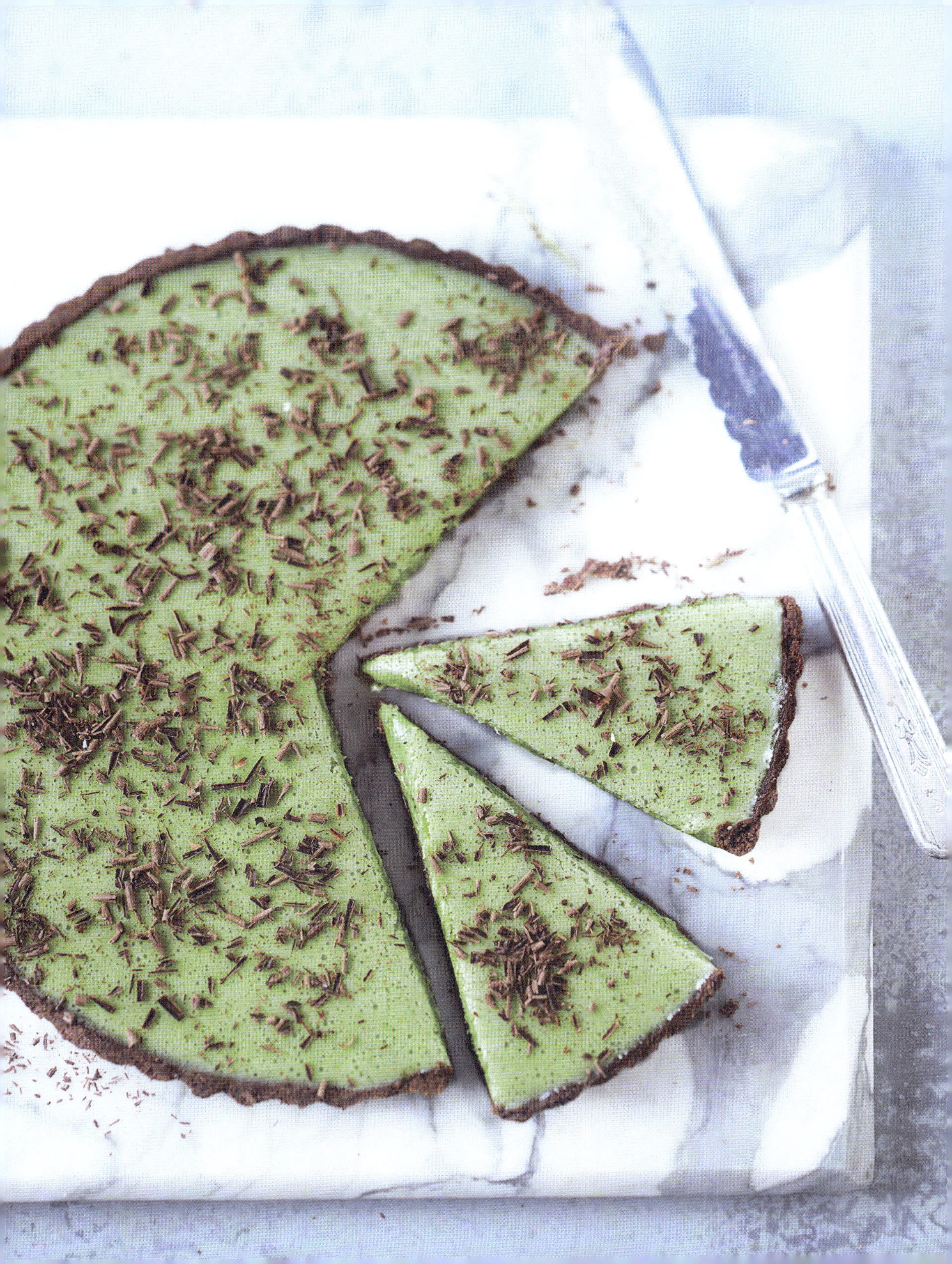

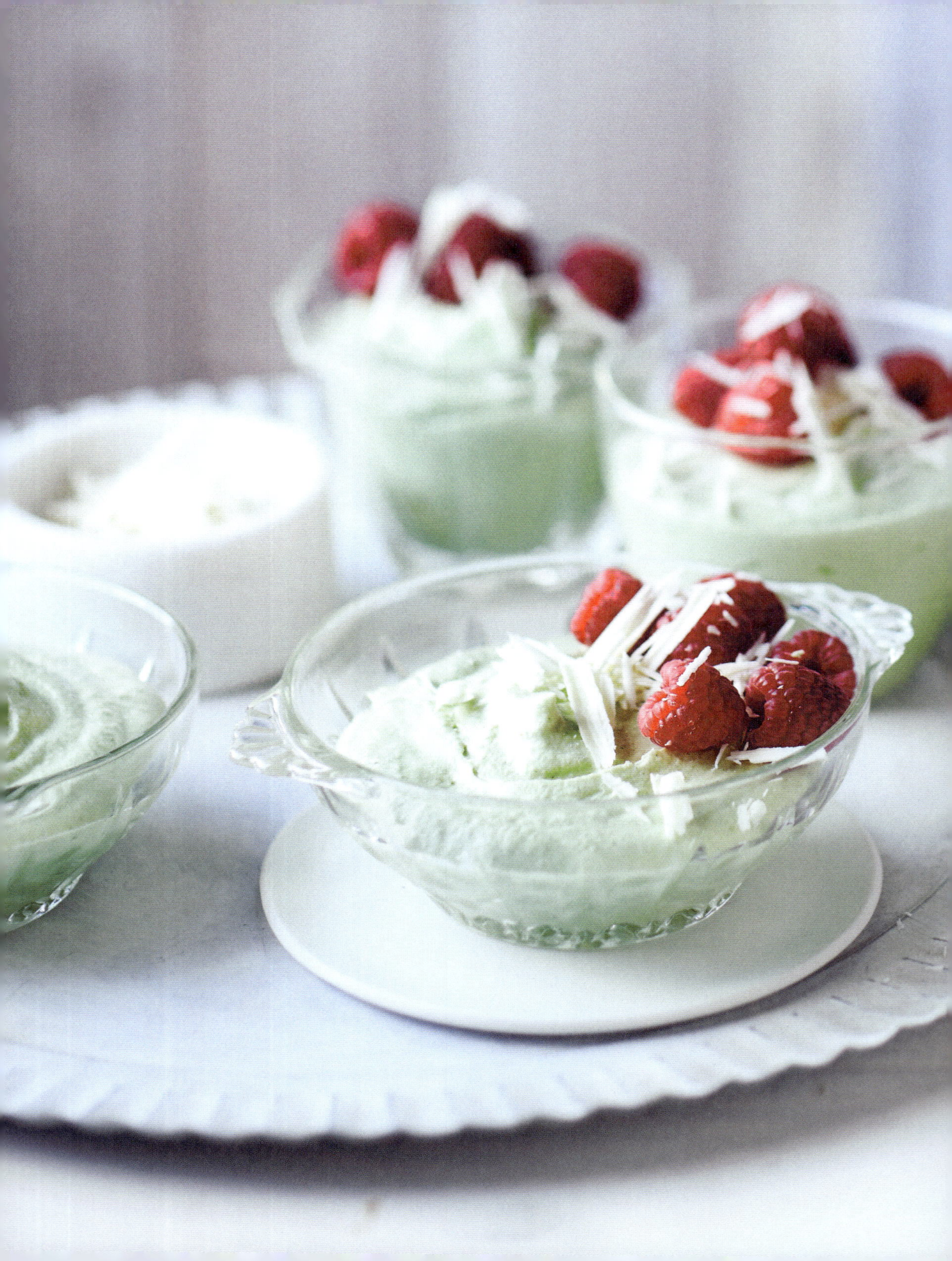

White chocolate matcha mousse

You just can't go wrong with the combination of white chocolate and matcha – these two ingredients taste sublime together and work brilliantly in this pretty dessert.

SERVES 6

2 tsp matcha powder
300ml (1¼ cups) double (heavy) cream
250g (9oz) white chocolate, roughly chopped
125ml (½ cup) milk
few drops of vanilla extract
3 egg whites
shaved white chocolate and fresh berries, to serve

1 Whisk the matcha powder with 3 tbsp cream in a heatproof bowl. When they are thoroughly combined and no lumps of matcha remain, add the chocolate and place the bowl over a saucepan of simmering water. Stir gently until the chocolate melts, then remove from the heat and stir in the milk.

2 In a clean bowl, whisk the remaining cream with the vanilla until it forms soft peaks.

3 In another clean, dry bowl, beat the egg whites until fluffy and they form stiff peaks.

4 With a spatula or metal spoon, gently fold the melted chocolate mixture into the beaten egg whites until thoroughly mixed. Next, fold in the whipped cream, as gently and lightly as possible.

5 Divide the mixture between six ramekin dishes and chill in the fridge for at least 2–3 hours until set.

6 Serve decorated with white chocolate shavings or curls and fresh raspberries, strawberries or redcurrants.

VARIATIONS

- Instead of vanilla, you could try using cardamom as a subtle flavouring. Remove the seeds from 6 pods and place with the milk in a small saucepan. Heat through gently and then bring to the boil. Remove from the heat and leave to infuse before straining and adding to the melted chocolate as above.
- Decorate the mousses by simply dusting with cocoa powder.

No-bake matcha freezer cake

Truly decadent, with a wonderful hit of matcha goodness, this tastes great with strawberry coulis, and why not add a scoop of matcha ice cream (see page 162)?

SERVES 6

300g (10oz) digestive biscuits (graham crackers)
125g (1 stick) butter
600ml (2½ cups) double (heavy) cream
1 tbsp matcha powder
500g (2¼ cups) mascarpone
grated zest of 1 lemon
80g (¾ cup) caster (superfine) sugar
450g (4 cups) fresh berries, e.g. raspberries or halved strawberries
125g (1 cup) hazelnuts, toasted and halved
dark chocolate curls or shards, to serve

FOR THE RASPBERRY COULIS

175g (1½ cups) raspberries
1 tbsp icing (confectioner's) sugar
juice of ½ lemon

1 Line the base of a 25cm (10in) loose-bottomed cake tin (pan) with baking parchment.

2 To make the biscuit base, crush the biscuits by placing them in a plastic bag and bashing them with a rolling pin, or pulse in a blender or food processor until they resemble breadcrumbs.

3 Melt the butter in a saucepan over a low heat and then stir in the crushed biscuits. Spoon into the lined tin and press down well with the back of a spoon to level the top. Chill in the fridge for 30 minutes.

4 Meanwhile, make the raspberry coulis. Blitz the raspberries in a food processor or blender until smooth. Add the icing sugar and pulse briefly. Pass through a sieve, discard any pips and stir in the lemon juice. Set aside.

5 In a clean bowl, whip the cream and matcha powder until thick and uniformly green. Add the mascarpone, lemon zest and sugar and fold in gently until thoroughly mixed and smooth. Then fold in the berries and hazelnuts.

6 Spoon the mixture into the tin, covering the biscuit base, and smooth the top. Wrap in aluminium foil and place in the freezer. Freeze for at least 5 hours.

7 When ready to serve, sprinkle the top of the cake with chocolate curls or shards. Allow the cake to stand at room temperature for about 15–20 minutes before removing from the tin and cutting into slices. Serve with a little pool of raspberry coulis.

VARIATIONS

- Vary the fruit and nuts: try blueberries, redcurrants or even peaches with flaked or nibbed almonds.
- Use gingernuts (gingersnaps) instead of digestive biscuits, or add a little ground cinnamon to the crumb and melted butter mixture.

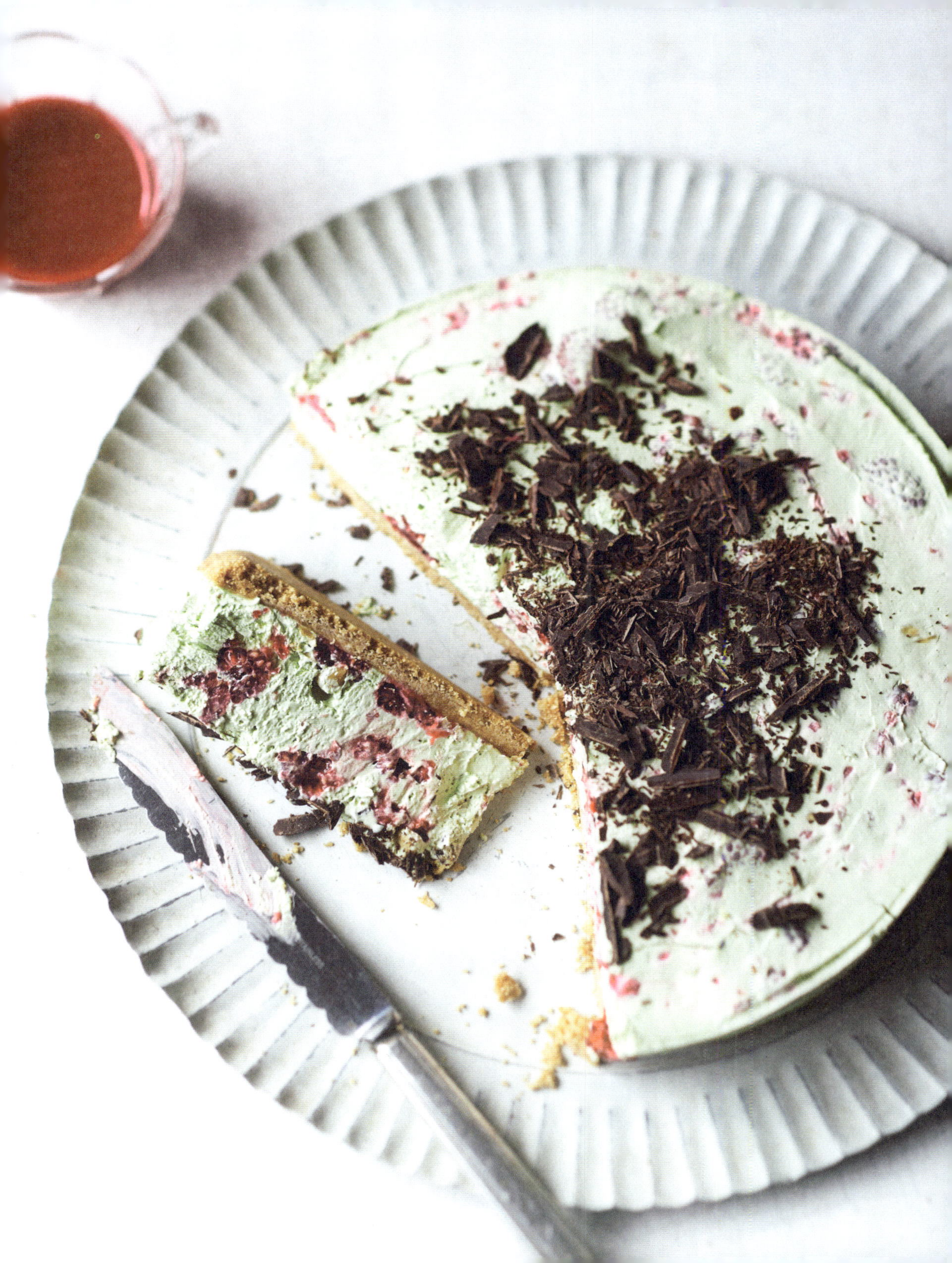

Choc chip and matcha ice cream

This gorgeously green ice cream is a real crowd-pleaser. To make a plain version just omit the grated chocolate – perfect with the Chocolate and matcha tart (see page 156).

SERVES 6

250ml (1 cup) milk
1 heaped tbsp matcha powder
6 egg yolks
150g (½ cup) caster (superfine) sugar
500ml (2 cups) double (heavy) cream
40g (1½oz) dark (bittersweet) chocolate (70% cocoa solids), coarsely grated

1 Heat the milk in a saucepan. Stir 2 tbsp warm milk (not too hot, nor too cold) into the matcha powder in a small bowl. Mix well to get rid of any lumps.

2 Beat the egg yolks and sugar together in a bowl until fluffy and light. Bring the milk to the boil and then whisk into the egg mixture. Pour it back into the warm saucepan and heat gently over a low heat, stirring all the time, until the custard thickens and coats the back of the spoon. Stir in the matcha mixture and set aside to cool.

3 Whip the cream until it forms soft peaks and gently fold it into the cooled matcha custard.

4 You can freeze this in an ice-cream maker, according to the manufacturer's instructions, and add the grated chocolate at the end.

5 Alternatively, pour the matcha ice cream mixture into a container, then cover and freeze for 3–4 hours until frozen softly and setting round the edges.

6 Remove from the freezer and transfer the ice cream to a food mixer or food processor and mix briefly to break up any ice crystals and make it slushy. Fold in the grated chocolate and spoon back into the container. Cover and freeze for a few hours or overnight until frozen.

7 Remove from the freezer about 15–20 minutes before serving to soften the ice cream slightly.

VARIATIONS

- Try using white instead of dark chocolate.
- For a minty version, add a dash of peppermint extract or steep some fresh mint leaves in the warm milk to add a subtle flavour and aroma.

Coconut and matcha ice cream

Making ice cream is so satisfying. Making green matcha ice cream is even more satisfying! This tastes simply amazing, and is perfect on a hot summer's day.

SERVES 4

1 x 400g (14oz) can coconut milk
1 tbsp cornflour (cornstarch)
1 tbsp matcha powder
85g (½ cup) caster (superfine) sugar
2 tbsp agave syrup or maple syrup
3 tbsp coconut cream
grated zest of 1 lime
toasted coconut flakes, to serve

1 Heat the coconut milk gently in a saucepan over a low heat. Put 4 tbsp of the warm milk in a small bowl and mix with the cornflour and matcha powder until smooth and lump-free.

2 Add the sugar to the saucepan and stir over a low heat until dissolved. Turn up the heat and as soon as it starts to boil, stir in the cornflour and matcha mixture. Reduce the heat and stir gently for 2–3 minutes until slightly thickened, creamy and smooth.

3 Remove from the heat and stir in the agave or maple syrup, coconut cream and lime zest. Set aside to cool.

4 Transfer to an ice-cream maker and follow the manufacturer's instructions.

5 Alternatively, spoon into a container, cover with a lid and freeze for 3–4 hours until frozen slightly and setting around the edges.

6 Remove from the freezer and transfer the ice cream to a food mixer or food processor and mix briefly to break up any ice crystals and make it slushy. Retun to the container, cover and freeze for a few hours or overnight until frozen. For really smooth ice cream, repeat the process again 3–4 hours later before freezing overnight.

7 Remove the ice cream from the freezer about 15–20 minutes before serving to soften it slightly. Serve in scoops sprinkled with toasted coconut flakes.

VARIATIONS

- Instead of lime zest, add a few drops of vanilla extract for flavouring.
- Sprinkle the ice cream with cacao nibs, pomegranate seeds or flaked (slivered) almonds.

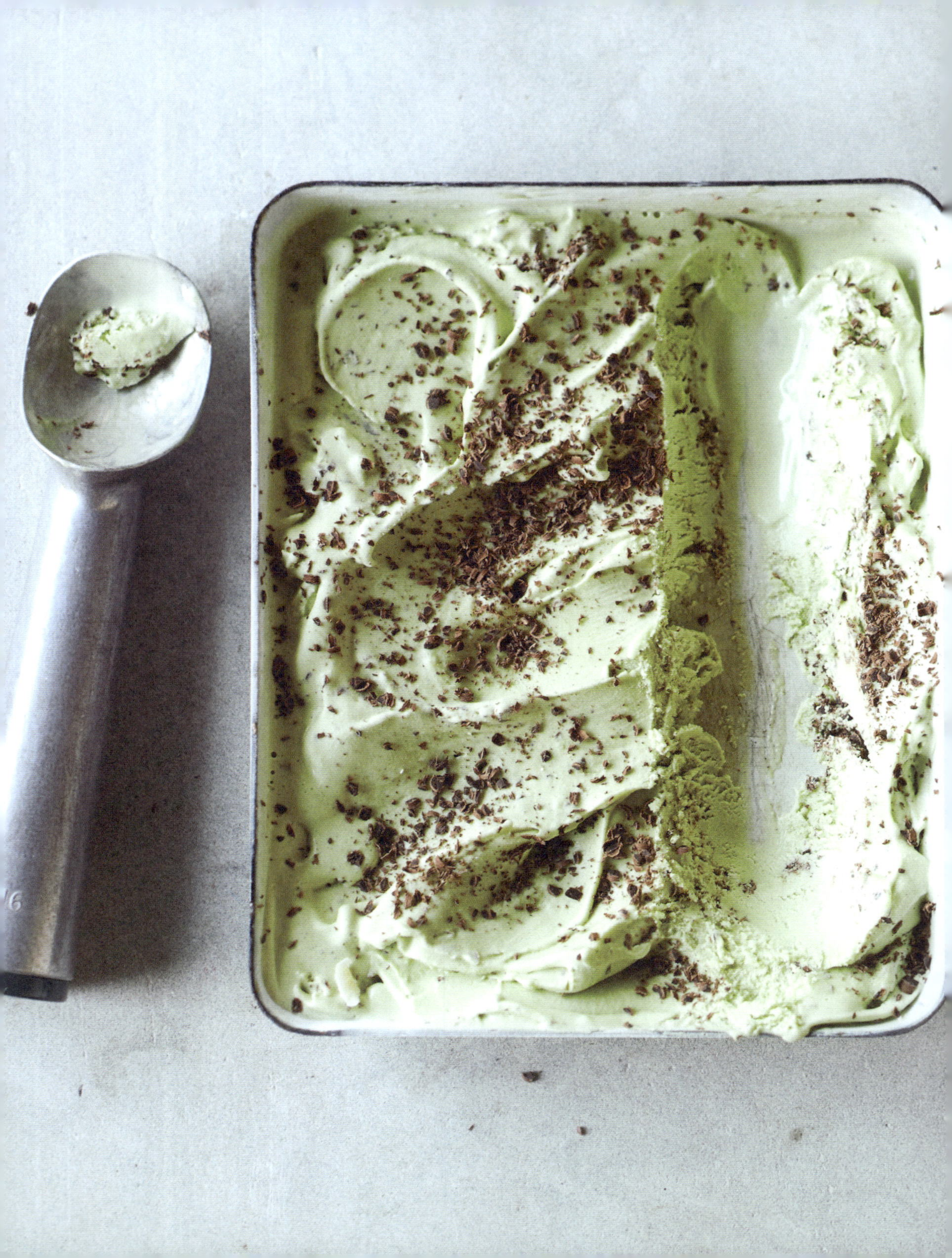

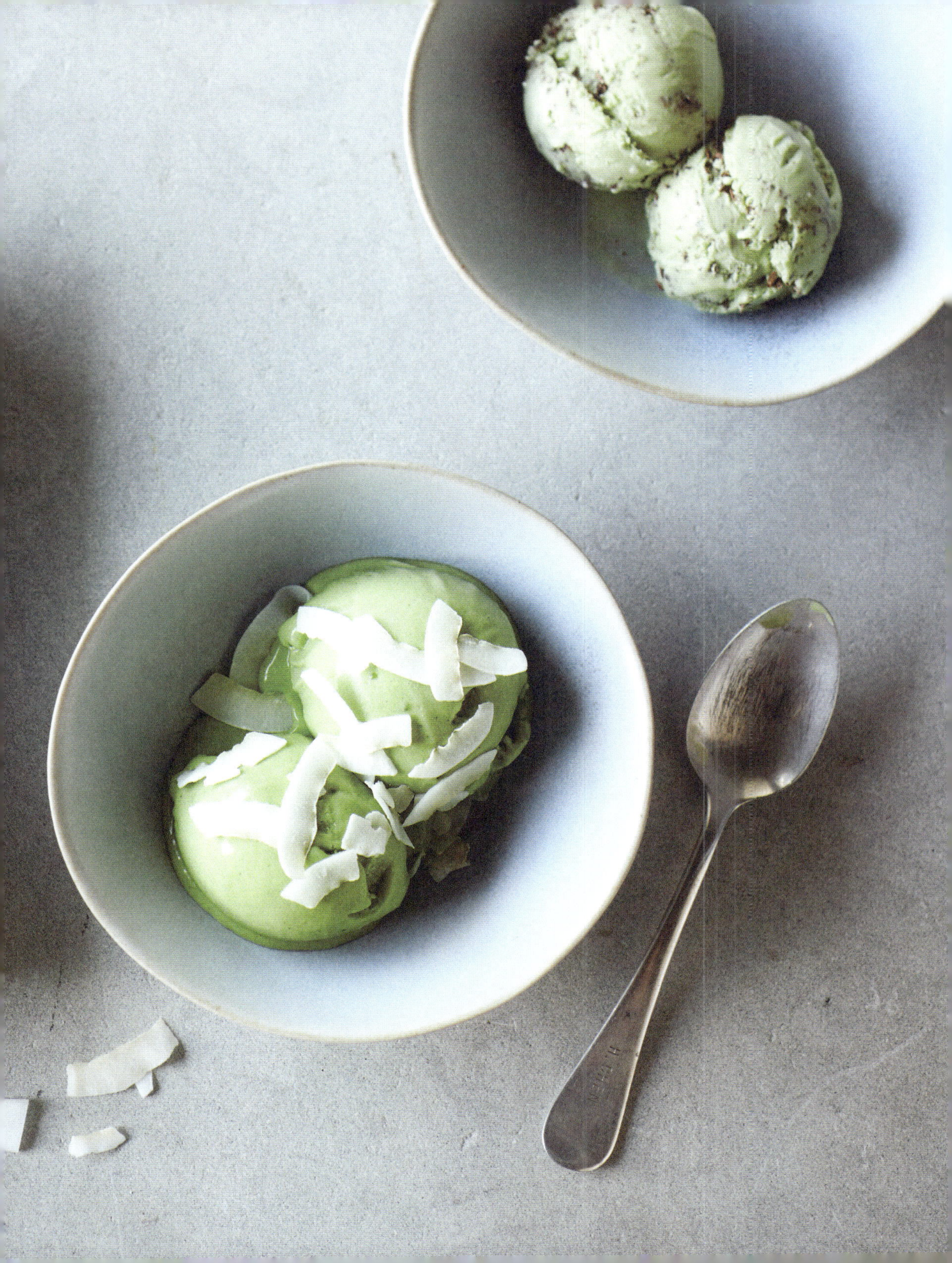

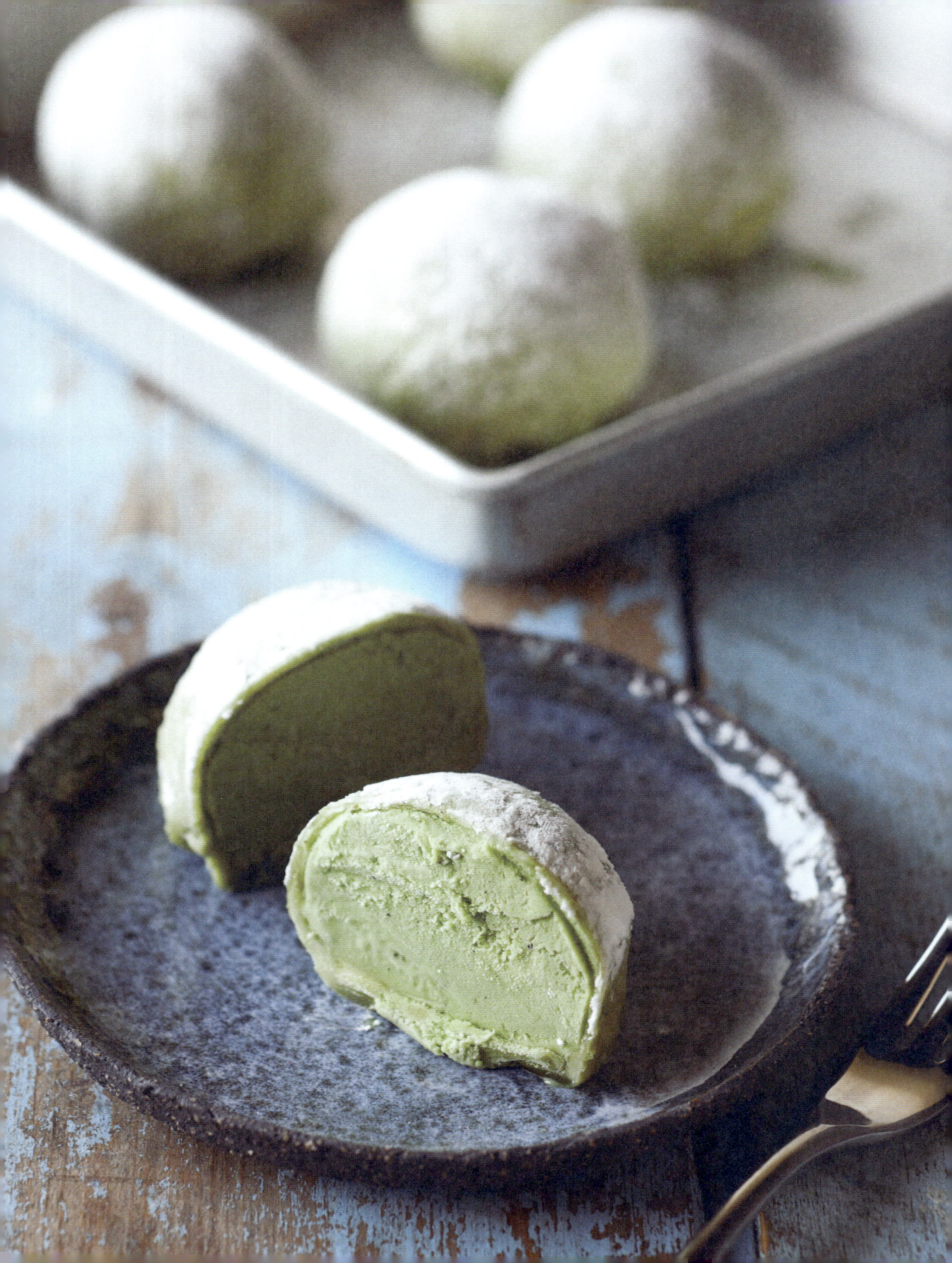

Matcha mochi ice cream balls

This is a wonderful, traditional Japanese sweet treat. Make your own matcha ice cream following the recipe on page 162 (omitting the chocolate) or page 163.

MAKES 9 MATCHA MOCHI BALLS

9 small scoops of matcha ice cream (see pages 162 or 163)
150g (1 cup) glutinous rice flour
pinch of salt
175ml (¾ cup) cold water
60g (¼ cup) caster (superfine) sugar
1 tsp matcha powder
cornflour (cornstarch), for dusting

1 Scoop the matcha ice cream into 9 paper baking cases (cupcake liners). Alternatively, line 9 cups of a cardboard egg carton with cling film (plastic wrap) and put a scoop into each cup. Cover the scoops with cling film and freeze for 2–3 hours until they are frozen solid.

2 To make the mochi dough, mix the rice flour, salt and water in a microwave-safe bowl. Add the sugar, stirring until smooth, and then whisk in the matcha powder. You should end up with a smooth mixture without any clumps of matcha.

3 Cover the bowl with cling film and microwave on high for 1 minute. Uncover the bowl and stir. Cover and microwave for 1 more minute, and then repeat this process again. If there's still some liquid left, keep microwaving for 30 seconds at a time until the dough is thick, gelatinous and sticky.

4 Dust a clean work surface with plenty of cornflour and place the ball of dough on top. Sprinkle with more cornflour and press the dough out with your hands or roll out with a rolling pin to a square, about 6mm (¼in) thick. Cut into 9 equal-sized squares and leave to cool.

5 Remove a frozen ice cream ball from the cling film and place on a cooled dough square. Quickly gather the dough around the ball to cover it completely, pinching the ends together neatly to seal it. Trim off and discard any excess dough. You need to work fast or the ice cream will melt. Cover the ball with cling film and replace in the paper case or egg carton and freeze immediately. Repeat this with the other 8 ice cream balls.

6 Freeze for about 2 hours until the matcha mochi are really frozen and firm. Remove from the freezer a few minutes before serving.

Matcha yoghurt ice lollies

As far as lollies (ice pops) go, 'there's plenty of good stuff packed into these refreshing treats, notably protein and calcium from the yoghurt, and not forgetting the polyphenol-packed matcha'. Just add summer sunshine for vitamin D!

MAKES 6 ICE LOLLIES

500g (2 cups) Greek yoghurt with honey
2 tsp matcha powder
few drops of vanilla extract

VARIATIONS

- For a dairy-free version use soya yoghurt.
- Try stirring some mochi pieces (see page 167), blueberries or small chunks of peeled, stoned (pitted) lychees into the yoghurt mixture before freezing.
- Instead of separating the yoghurt mixtures, mix everything together and then add a mashed ripe avocado together with 2–3 tbsp almond milk. Blend well, spoon into the moulds and freeze as above.

1 Whisk together one-fifth of the Greek yoghurt with the matcha powder until smooth, lump-free and uniformly coloured.

2 In another bowl, add the vanilla extract to the remaining yoghurt.

3 Divide the matcha yoghurt mixture between 6 ice lolly (pop) moulds and top with the remaining vanilla yoghurt mixture.

4 Insert a wooden lolly stick into the centre of each lolly and freeze for a few hours or overnight until well frozen.

5 To serve, hold the moulds under cold running water and then ease out the frozen lollies.

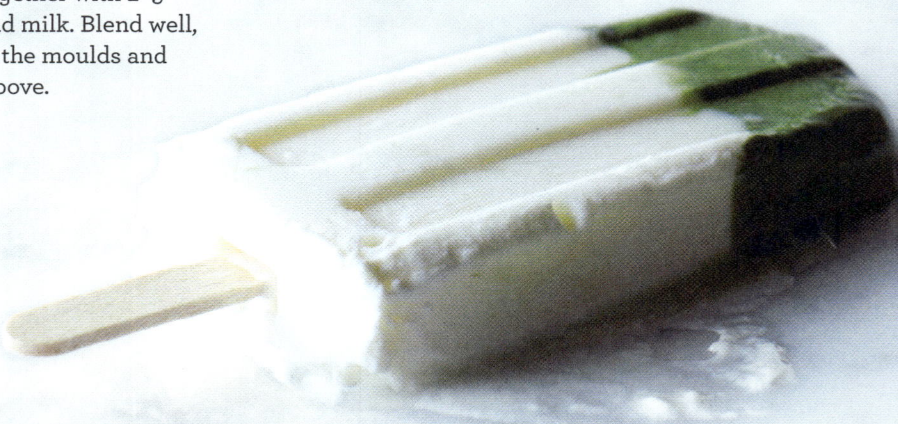

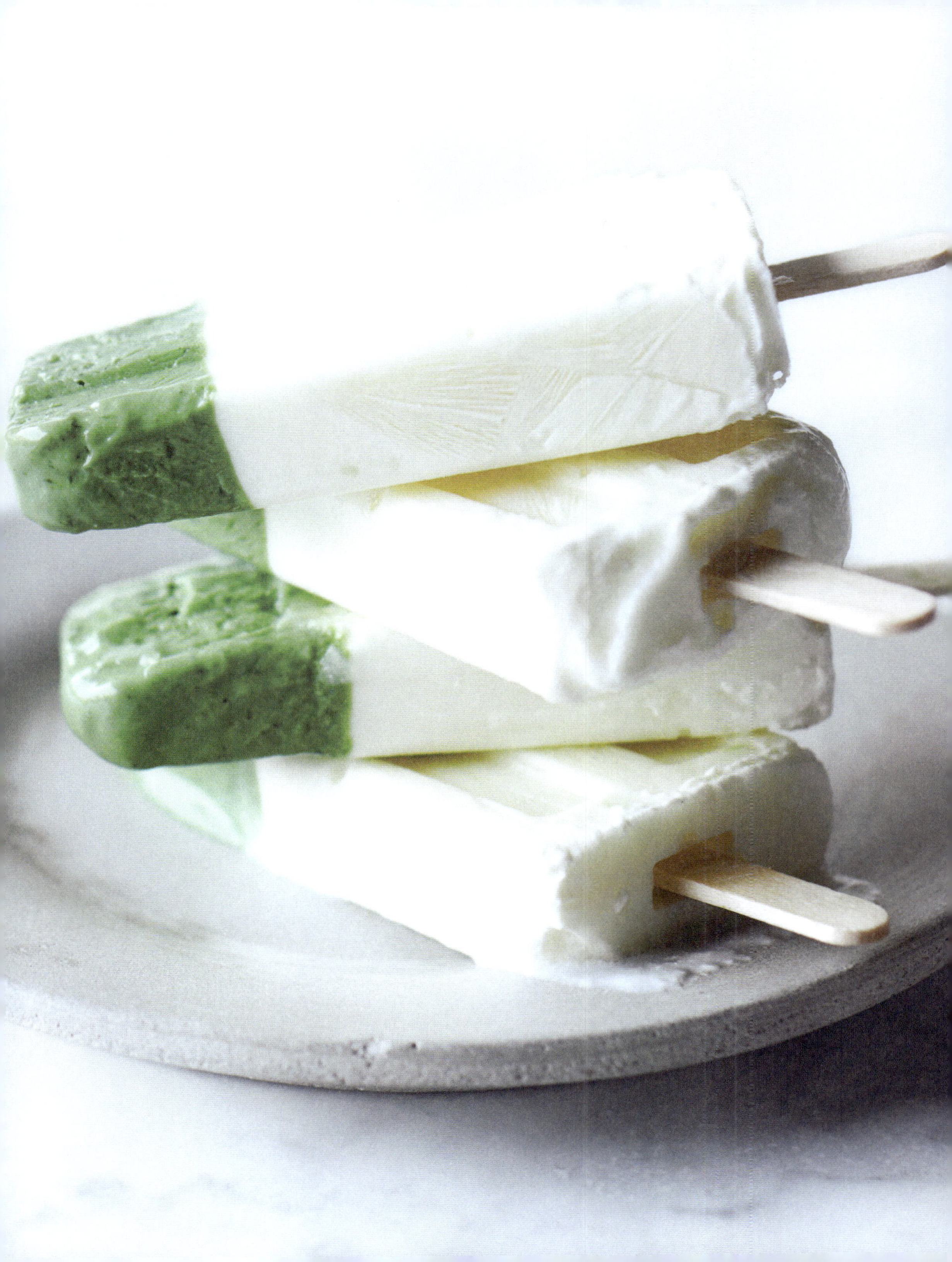

INDEX

A
ageing 36
Akatsuki-no-chaji 19
alcohol, matcha 47
almond milk: almond matcha latte 62
chia seed and matcha power pots 94
dairy-free almond and matcha frappé 65
dairy-free smoothie 76
matcha overnight oats 79
almonds: matcha macarons 144–7
amino acids 25, 26, 34, 36
antioxidants 36, 40
apple juice: beautiful berry juice 60
glorious green juice 60
peach and apple juice 60
apples: the green smoothie 76
aracha 25, 27
Australia 50
avocados: matcha guacamole 128

B
bananas: coconut breakfast smoothie 77
glorious green juice 60
matcha banana bread 103
matcha breakfast muffins 84
vanilla matcha milkshake 66
Bancha tea 25
beef: steak and noodle salad with matcha dressing 117
beer, matcha 46
berries: beautiful berry juice 60
matcha granola with berries 74
no-bake matcha freezer cake 148
biscuits: mini matcha cheesecakes 154
no-bake matcha freezer cake 160
raisin, oat and matcha cookies 148
black tea 9, 22, 38
blondies, matcha 140
blood pressure 38
blood sugar 39
blueberry compote, matcha yoghurt with 81
Bocha 25
body composition 39
bone health 39
broccoli: matcha poached salmon, broccoli and chickpea salad 112
Buddhism 8, 9, 11, 37, 44

C
caffeine 25, 36, 41
cakes: chocolate layer cake with matcha icing 134
coconut and matcha cupcakes 139
matcha banana bread 103
matcha blondies 140
calorie burning 36
Camellia sinensis 22
Canada 50
cancer 36, 38
cardiovascular disease 38
catechins 36, 38–9, 40, 41
ceremonies, tea 9, 11, 12, 13, 14, 15, 16, 17, 18, 19, 28, 29, 44, 48, 49
Cha-no-yu 11, 12, 13
chabako 16
Chado 12–19
chaki 16
champagne: mint fizz cocktail 70
chanoyugama 13, 17
Chanyuan Qinggi 11
chasen 16
chashaku 16
chawan 16
cheesecakes, mini matcha 154
chia seed and matcha power pots 94
chicken: chicken, turmeric, matcha and pepper casserole 126
Mexican chicken with matcha guacamole 128
chickpeas: matcha poached salmon, broccoli and chickpea salad 112
chilli dressing, matcha 110
China 8, 10, 11, 22, 29, 30
chlorophyll 25, 34
chocolate: choc chip and matcha ice cream 162
chocolate and matcha tart 156
chocolate layer cake with matcha icing 134
matcha banana bread 103
matcha blondies 140
white chocolate and matcha milkshake 66
white chocolate matcha latte 62
white chocolate matcha mousse 159

cholesterol 38, 79
cocktails, matcha 70
coconut: raw matcha coconut
fudge bites 106
coconut ice cream: matcha
coconut teashake 65
coconut milk: coconut and
matcha cupcakes 139
coconut and matcha ice
cream 163
coconut breakfast
smoothie 77
the green smoothie 76
matcha coconut teashake 65
concentration 36
cookies, raisin, oat and
matcha 148
coulis, raspberry 160
cream cheese: mini matcha
cheesecakes 154
crisps, matcha 47
croissants, matcha 86–7
cupcakes, coconut and
matcha 139
curry, matcha Thai green 125

D
dairy-free almond and matcha
frappé 65
dairy-free smoothie 76
dates: raw sticky date and
matcha bars 100
diabetes 39
dora 17
doughnuts, matcha ring 142
dressings, matcha 110, 112, 114,
117, 123
drinks 46, 54–5, 60–70

E
EGCG (epigallocatechin
gallate) 36, 38, 40, 41
eggs: choc chip and matcha
ice cream 150
matcha eggs Florentine 82
matcha soufflés 140
Eisai, Myoan 10, 12, 13
energy 36–7
English muffins: matcha eggs
Florentine 82
equipment 18

F
fat oxidization 36
flavonoids 6, 36
flax seeds: raw sticky date and
matcha bars 100
focus 36–7
frappé, dairy-free almond and
matcha 64
freezer cake, no-bake matcha 160
fudge bites, raw matcha
coconut 106
fukumi 27

G
Genmaicha 24–5
Germany 50
ginger ale: citrus mocktail 70
gnocchi, matcha 118
Goggins, Aidan 38–41
Grand Marnier: green
martini 70
granola: matcha granola with
berries 82
green beans, wasabi tuna with
matcha 123
green beer 46
green martini 70
green tea 8–9, 24–9, 34, 36–41
green tea extract 36
health benefits 36–41
history of 8–11
Japanese green tea 24–5
see also matcha
guacamole, matcha 128
Gyokuro Tamahomare 25

H
hachi 17
hachiju-hachiya 25, 26
harvesting of tea 26
Hatsugama 19
hazelnut milk: hazelnut and
vanilla smoothie 74
hazelnuts: no-bake matcha
freezer cake 160
health benefits 32–41
heart health 38
history of matcha 6–11
Hojicha 25
hollandaise sauce, matcha 90
Hong Kong 50

I
ice cream: choc chip and
matcha ice cream 162
coconut and matcha ice
cream 163
matcha ice cream 46
matcha mochi ice cream
balls 167
ice lollies, matcha yoghurt 168
iced tea, matcha mint 69
ichi-go ichi-e 13
icings: coconut matcha icing 139
matcha buttercream 144–7
matcha icing 134
Ikeda, Kikunae 45

J
Japan 8–11, 29, 30–1, 46, 48–9
green teas 24–5
history of matcha 6–11
matcha and Japanese
cuisine 44
matcha tea production
20–31
tea ceremonies 9, 11, 12, 13,
14, 15, 16, 17, 18, 19, 28, 29,
44, 48, 49

jikagise 25, 26
jikyaki 18
Joo, Takeno 9
juices 60

K

kale: glorious green juice 60
  the green smoothie 76
kama 13, 17
Kuchikiri-no-chaji 19
Kukai 10
Kukicha 25
kuromoji 17
kyaku 19

L

lattes 46, 52
lemon sorbet: citrus
  mocktail 70
lemonade, matcha 68
L-theanine 9, 25, 26, 36, 41

M

macarons, matcha 144–7
marshmallows, matcha 104–5
martini, green 70
mascarpone: no-bake matcha
  freezer cake 160
matcha 24
  choosing, storing and
    preparing 54–5
  differences between matcha
    and green tea 28
  drinking matcha 44
  as a food ingredient 44–7
  grades 26–7
  health benefits 32–41
  history of 6–11
  making the traditional way 55
  the matcha challenge 56
  optimizing your matcha
    intake 41
  production 10–11, 20–31
  taste 22, 24–5, 26, 28, 44–5, 54
Matten, Glen 38–41
Mexican chicken with matcha
  guacamole 128
milk: white chocolate matcha
  latte 62
  milkshakes: vanilla matcha
    milkshake 66
  white chocolate and matcha
    milkshake 66
mint: citrus mocktail 70
  matcha mint iced tea 69
  mint fizz cocktail 70
mousse, white chocolate
  matcha 159
muffins, matcha breakfast
  84
mushrooms: shiitake, pak
  choi and matcha teriyaki
  stir-fry 120
Myoe 10

N

Nagatani, Soen 10, 24
Nagori-no-Chaji 19
neriko 17
nervous system 41
Nishio 28, 29, 30
no-bake matcha freezer
  cake 160
Nobunaga, Oda 9
noodles: matcha Thai green
  curry 125
steak and noodle salad 117
stir-fried pork and matcha
  soba noodles 130

O

oats: matcha breakfast
  muffins 84
matcha granola with
  berries 82
matcha overnight oats 79
raisin, oat and matcha
  cookies 148
raw sticky date and matcha
  bars 100
oolong tea 9, 22
osteoporosis 39

P

pak choi: shiitake, pak choi
  and matcha teriyaki stir-fry
  120
pancakes, matcha 88
pastry: chocolate pastry 156
  matcha pastries 46
peaches: chia seed and matcha
  power pots 94
  peach and apple juice 60
peanut butter: prawn satay
  salad 114
peanuts: steak and noodle
  salad 117
pears: the green smoothie 76
pistachios: matcha pistachio
  protein balls 99
plucking 22
polyphenols 36, 60
popcorn tea 25
pork: stir-fried pork and
  matcha soba noodles 130
power pots, chia seed and
  matcha 94
prawns: matcha Thai green
  curry with king prawns 125
prawn satay salad 114
pretzels, matcha 96
producers of matcha 30–1
production of matcha 20–31, 34
protein balls, matcha
  pistachio 99
pu-erh 9

Q

quinoa salad with matcha
  chilli dressing 110

R

raisin, oat and matcha cookies 148
raspberry coulis 160
raw matcha coconut fudge bites 106
raw sticky date and matcha bars 100
red matcha 29
red tea 9
Rikyu, Sen no 9, 11, 13
Rooibos 29
Rwanda 22

S

Sado 12–19
Saga 10
Saicho 10
salads: matcha poached salmon, broccoli and chickpea salad 112
  prawn satay salad with matcha dressing 114
  quinoa salad with matcha chilli dressing 110
  steak and noodle salad with matcha dressing 117
salmon: matcha poached salmon, broccoli and chickpea salad 112
Samurai class 9
satay salad, prawn 114
Sencha 12, 24–5
shokyaku 18
Shuko, Murato 9
Singapore 50
Sirtfoods 40
sirtuins 40
skin damage 36
smoothies 74–7
Sojun, Ikkyu 9
soufflés, matcha 152
spinach: matcha eggs Florentine 90
steaming 8, 11, 24, 26
stir-fries: shiitake, pak choi and matcha teriyaki stir-fry 120
  stir-fried pork and matcha soba noodles 130
storing matcha 54
Swiss roll, matcha 136

T

Taiwan 22
Tana 10, 25, 26
tart, chocolate and matcha 156
tea 12–13, 22–5
  Japanese tea ceremonies 9, 11, 12, 13, 14, 15, 16, 17, 18, 19, 28, 29, 44, 48, 49
  matcha mint iced tea 69
  see also green tea; white tea, etc
tea houses 14, 48–9
tea masters 9
teashake, matcha coconut 65
tencha 25, 27, 30
tenmoku 17
teriyaki: shiitake, pak choi and matcha teriyaki stir-fry 120
Thai green curry with king prawns 125
theanine 9, 25, 26, 36, 41
thermogenesis 36
toast, matcha on 47
tuna: wasabi tuna with matcha green beans 123
twig tea 25

U

Uji 10, 24, 28, 29, 30, 47
umami flavour 24, 26, 28, 45, 54
UK 51
USA 51

V

vanilla: hazelnut and vanilla smoothie 74
  vanilla matcha milkshake 66
vodka: green martini 70

W

walnuts: matcha breakfast muffins 84
wasabi tuna with matcha green beans 123
Way of Tea 9, 12–19
weight 39
white tea 22, 29

Y

yoghurt: chia seed and matcha power pots 94
  hazelnut and vanilla smoothie 74
  matcha granola with berries 82
  matcha yoghurt ice lollies 168
  matcha yoghurt with blueberry compote 81

ACKNOWLEDGEMENTS

We would like to thank the teapigs team for making matcha 'a thing'. Big thanks to **Sofia, Charlotte L, Charlotte N** and **Anna** for working so hard on the delicious matcha recipes (and eating the delicious matcha products!). Thanks also to all our lovely trade customers who have supported the growth of this magical green tea.

PICTURE CREDITS

The publisher would like to thank the following sources for their kind permission to reproduce the photographs in this book: **Page 2** Getty Images/Westend61; **4** Jacqui Small; **6–7** Jacqui Small; **10** (b) Alamy Stock Photo/ Glasshouse Images; **12** (c) Getty Images/ARO @ PHOTOGRAPHY; **14** (b) Alamy Stock Photo/Oote Boe Ph; **17** NewAfrica/Shutterstock; **20–1** Jacqui Small; **22** (bl) Alamy Stock Photo/Japan Stock Photography; **23** Alamy Stock Photo/PhotoAlto sas; **24** (cl) 123rf/Diana Taliun; **24** (cr) 123rf/Baramee Thaweesombat; **24** (br) 123rf/sahua; **25** (cl, bl and cr) 123rf/sahua; **31**(t) Alamy Stock Photo/epa european pressphoto agency b.v; **31** (bl) Getty Images/ Sankei/Contributor; **31** (br) Alamy Stock Photo/epa european pressphoto agency b.v; **32–3** teapigs; **34** Jacqui Small; **35** Alamy Stock Photo/ PhotoCuisine; **37** Jacqui Small; **42–3** Jacqui Small; **45** (tl) Jacqui Small; **45** (bc) iStock/hirenman69; **45** (br) iStock/Joey333; **47** (tl) Shutterstock/Selinofoto; **47** (tr) Shutterstock/Elena Demyanko; **47** (bl) 123rf/Dontree Malaimarn; **47** (br) Jacqui Small; **49** Tondaya, Kyoto; **51** Winstons Coffee, Hong Kong; **52–3** Jacqui Small; **55** iStock /kalasek; all photos pages **58–169** Jacqui Small, with the exception of pages **77** Master Q/Shutterstock; and **175** teapigs.

REFERENCES

Page 36:

1. Yusuf, Irby, Katiyar and Elmets. 'Photoprotective effects of green tea polyphenols', *Photodermatol Photoimmunol Photomed* (2007): 23: 48–56.

Pages 38–9:

1. Zheng, Jusheng, et al. 'Green tea and black tea consumption and prostate cancer risk: an exploratory meta-analysis of observational studies.' *Nutrition and cancer* 63.5 (2011): 663–672.

2. Kang, Hyunseok, et al. 'Green tea consumption and stomach cancer risk: a meta-analysis.' *Epidemiology and health* 32 (2010): e2010001.

3. Tang, Naping, et al. 'Green tea, black tea consumption and risk of lung cancer: a meta-analysis.' *Lung cancer* 65.3 (2009): 274–283.

4. Ogunleye, Adeyemi A., Fei Xue, and Karin B. Michels. 'Green tea consumption and breast cancer risk or recurrence: a meta-analysis.' *Breast cancer research and treatment* 119.2 (2010): 477–484.

5. Onakpoya, I., et al. 'The effect of green tea on blood pressure and lipid profile: A systematic review and meta-analysis of randomized clinical trials.' *Nutrition, Metabolism and Cardiovascular Diseases* 24.8 (2014): 823–836.

6. Kuriyama, Shinichi, et al. 'Green tea consumption and mortality due to cardiovascular disease, cancer, and all causes in Japan: the Ohsaki study.' *Jama* 296.10 (2006): 1255–1265.

7. Liu, Kai, et al. 'Effect of green tea on glucose control and insulin sensitivity: a meta-analysis of 17 randomized controlled trials.' *The American journal of clinical nutrition* 98.2 (2013): 340–348.

8. Jing, Yali, et al. 'Tea consumption and risk of type 2 diabetes: a meta-analysis of cohort studies.' *Journal of general internal medicine* 24.5 (2009): 557–562.

9. Yang, Jian, et al. 'Tea consumption and risk of type 2 diabetes mellitus: a systematic review and meta-analysis update.' *BMJ* open 4.7 (2014): e005632.

10. Shen, Chwan-Li, Ming-Chien Chyu, and Jia-Sheng Wang. 'Tea and bone health: steps forward in translational nutrition.' *The American journal of clinical nutrition* 98.6 (2013): 1694S–1699S.

11. Wu, ChihHsing, et al. 'Relationship among habitual tea consumption, percent body fat, and body fat distribution.' *Obesity research* 11.9 (2003): 1088–1095.

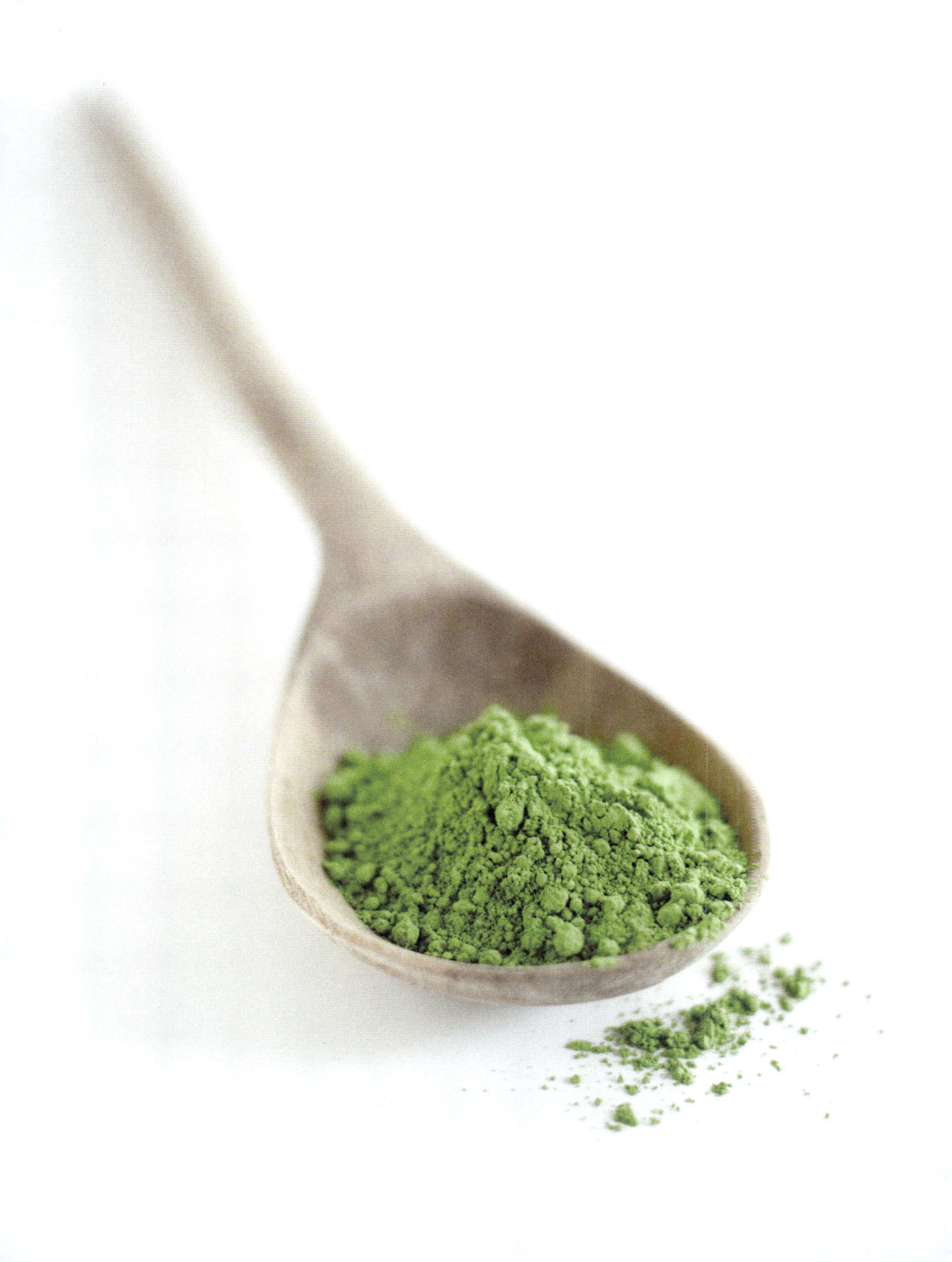

Quarto

First published in 2016 by Jaqui Small LLP
an imprint of The Quarto Group.
One Triptych Place, London, SE1 9SH,
United Kingdom
T (0)20 7700 9000
www.Quarto.com

This revised edition published in 2026 by White Lion Publishing

EEA Representation, WTS Tax d.o.o., Žanova ulica 3, 4000 Kranj, Slovenia
www.wts-tax.si

A catalogue record for this book is available from the British Library.

ISBN 978-1-80570-243-6
Ebook ISBN 978-1-91112-709-3

10 9 8 7 6 5 4 3 2 1

Design by Ginny Zeal
Illustrations by Emma Cobb
Food photography by David Munns
Written by Louise Cheadle and Nick Kilby

Publisher: Jessica Axe
Project Editor: Melissa Hookway
Senior Designer: Renata Latipova
Senior Production Controller: Rohana Yusof

Printed in Malaysia PC122025

FSC www.fsc.org MIX Paper | Supporting responsible forestry FSC® C007207